Disease and Its Causes

by William Thomas Councilman

PREFACE

In this little volume the author has endeavored to portray disease as life under conditions which differ from the usual. Life embraces much that is unknown and in so far as disease is a condition of living things it too presents many problems which are insoluble with our present knowledge. Fifty years ago the extent of the unknown, and at that time insoluble questions of disease, was much greater than at present, and the problems now are in many ways different from those in the past. No attempt has been made to simplify the subject by the presentation of theories as facts.

The limitation as to space has prevented as full a consideration of the subject as would be desirable for clearness, but a fair division into the general and concrete phases of disease has been attempted. Necessarily most attention has been given to the infectious diseases and their causes. This not only because these diseases are the most important but they are also the best known and give the simplest illustrations. The space given to the infectious diseases has allowed a merely cursory description of the organic diseases and such subjects as insanity and heredity. Of the organic diseases most space has been devoted to disease of the heart. There is slight consideration of the environment and social conditions as causes of disease.

Very few authors are mentioned in the text and no bibliography is given. There is lack of literature dealing with the general aspects of disease; the book moreover is not written for physicians, and the list of investigators from whose work the knowledge of disease has been derived would be too long to cite.

It has been assumed that the reader has some familiarity with elementary anatomy and physiology, and these subjects have been considered only as much as is necessary to set the scene for the drama. I am indebted to my friend, Mr. W. R. Thayer, for patiently enduring the reading of the manuscript and for many suggestions as to phrasing.

CONTENTS

CHAPTER

CHAPTER I

CHAPTER II

CHAPTER III

RELATION BETWEEN INSANITY AND CRIMINALITY.--ALCOHOLISM AND SYPHILIS FREQUENT CAUSES OF INSANITY.--THE DIRECT AND INDIRECT CAUSES OF NERVOUS DISEASES.--THE RELATION BETWEEN SOCIAL LIFE AND NERVOUS DISEASES.--FUNCTIONAL AND ORGANIC DISEASE.--NEURASTHENIA

CHAPTER XII

THE RAPID DEVELOPMENT OF MEDICINE IN THE LAST FIFTY YEARS.--THE INFLUENCE OF DARWIN.--PREVENTIVE MEDICINE.--THE DISSEMINATION OF MEDICAL KNOWLEDGE.--THE DEVELOPMENT OF CONDITIONS IN RECENT YEARS WHICH ACT AS FACTORS OF DISEASE.--FACTORY LIFE.--URBAN LIFE.-- THE INCREASE OF COMMUNICATION BETWEEN PEOPLES.--THE INTRODUCTION OF PLANT PARASITES.--THE INCREASE IN ASYLUM LIFE.-- INFANT MORTALITY.--WEALTH AND POVERTY AS FACTORS IN DISEASE

GLOSSARY

DISEASE AND ITS CAUSES

CHAPTER I

DEFINITION OF DISEASE.--CHARACTERISTICS OF LIVING MATTER.--CELLS AS THE LIVING UNITS.--AMOEBA AS TYPE OF A UNICELLULAR ANIMAL.--THE RELATION OF LIVING MATTER TO THE ENVIRONMENT.--CAPACITY OF ADAPTATION TO THE ENVIRONMENT SHOWN BY LIVING MATTER-- INDIVIDUALITY OF LIVING MATTER.--THE CAUSES OF DISEASE.--EXTRINSIC.-- THE RELATION OF THE HUMAN BODY TO THE ENVIRONMENT.--THE SURFACES OF THE BODY.--THE INCREASE OF SURFACE BY GLAND FORMATION.- -THE REAL INTERIOR OF THE BODY REPRESENTED BY THE VARIOUS STRUCTURES PLACED BETWEEN THE SURFACES.--THE FLUIDS OF THE BODY.-- THE NERVOUS SYSTEM.--THE HEART AND BLOOD-VESSELS.--THE CELLS OF THE BLOOD.--THE DUCTLESS GLANDS.

There is great difficulty, in the case of a subject so large and complex as is disease, in giving a definition which will be accurate and comprehensive. Disease may be defined as "A change produced in living things in consequence of which they are no longer in harmony with their environment." It is evident that this conception of disease is inseparable from the idea of life, since only a living thing can become diseased. In any dead body there has been a preexisting disease or injury, and, in consequence of the change produced, that particular form of activity which constitutes life has ceased. Changes such as putrefaction take place in the dead body, but they are changes which would take place in any mass similarly constituted, and are not influenced by the fact that the mass was once living. Disease may also be thought of as the negation of the normal. There is, however, in living things no definite type for the normal. An ideal normal type may be constructed by taking the average of a large number of individuals; but any single individual of the group will, to a greater or less extent, depart from it. No two individuals have been found in whom all the Bertillon measurements agree. Disease has reference to the individual; conditions which in one individual would be regarded as disease need not be so regarded in another. Comparisons between health and disease, the normal and the abnormal, must be made not between the ideal normal and abnormal, but between what constitutes the normal or usual and the abnormal in a particular individual.

The conception of disease is so inseparably associated with that of life that a brief review of the structure and properties of living things is necessary for the comprehension of the definition which has been given. Living matter is subject to the laws which govern matter, and like matter of any other sort it is composed of atoms and molecules. There is no force inherent in living matter, no vital force independent of and differing from the cosmic forces; the energy which living matter gives off is counterbalanced by the energy which it receives. It undergoes constant change, and there is constant interchange with the environment. The molecules which compose it are constantly undergoing change in their number, kind and arrangement. Atom groups as decomposition products are constantly given off from it, and in return it receives from without other atom groups with which it regenerates its substance or increases in amount. All definitions of life convey this idea of activity. Herbert Spencer says, "Life is the continuous adjustment of internal relations to external conditions." The molecules of the substances forming the living material are large, complex and unstable, and as such they constantly tend to pass from the complex to the simple, from unstable to stable equilibrium. The elementary substances which form living material are known, but it has hitherto not been found possible artificially so to combine these substances that the resulting mass will exhibit those activities which we call the phenomena of life. The distinction between living and nonliving matter is manifest only when the sum of the activities of the living matter is considered; any single phenomenon of the living may appear also in the non-living material. Probably the most distinguishing criterion of living matter is found in its individuality, which undoubtedly depends upon differences in structure, whether physical or chemical, between the different units.

Certain conditions are essential for the continued existence of living matter. It must be surrounded by a fluid or semi-fluid medium in order that there may be easy interchange with the environment. It must constantly receive from the outside a supply of energy in the form of food, and substances formed as the result of the intracellular chemical activity must be removed. In the case of many animals it seems as though the necessity of a fluid environment for living matter did not apply, for the superficial cells of the skin have no fluid around them; these cells, however, are dead, and serve merely a mechanical or protective purpose. All the living cells of the skin and all the cells beneath this have fluid around them.

Living matter occurs always in the form of small masses called "cells," which are the living units. The cells vary in form, structure and size, some being so large that they can be seen with the naked eye, while others are so small that they cannot be distinctly seen with the highest power of the microscope. The living thing or organism may be composed of a single cell or, in the case of the higher animals and plants, may be formed of great numbers of cells, those of a similar character being combined in masses to form organs such as the liver and brain.

In each cell there is a differentiated area constituting a special structure, the nucleus, which contains a peculiar material called "chromatin." The nucleus has chiefly to do with the multiplication of the cell and contains the factors which determine heredity. The mass outside of the nucleus is termed "cytoplasm," and this may be homogeneous in appearance or may contain granules. On the outside there is a more or less definite cell membrane. It is generally believed that the cell material has a semi-fluid or gelatinous consistency and is contained within an intracellular meshwork. It is an extraordinarily complex mass, whether regarded from a chemical or physical point of view. (Fig. 1.)

[Illustration: FIG. 1.--DIAGRAM OF CELL. 1. Cell membrane. 2. Cell substance or cytoplasm. 3. Nucleus. 4. Nuclear membrane. 5. Nucleolus.]

A simple conception of health and disease can be arrived at by the study of these conditions in a unicellular animal directly under a microscope, the animal being placed on a glass slide. For this purpose a small organism called "Amoeba" (Fig. 2), which is commonly present in freshwater ponds, may be used. This appears as a small mass, seemingly of gelatinous consistency with a clear outline, the exterior part homogeneous, the interior granular. The nucleus, which is seen with difficulty, appears as a small vesicle in the interior. Many amoeba show also in the interior a small clear space, the contractile vesicle which alternately contracts and expands, through which action the movement of the intracellular fluid is facilitated and waste products removed. The interior granules often change their position, showing that there is motion within the mass. The amoeba slowly moves along the surface of the glass by the extension of blunt processes formed from the clear outer portion which adhere to the surface and into which the interior granular mass flows. This movement does not take place by chance, but in definite directions, and may be influenced. The amoeba will move towards certain substances which may be placed in the fluid around it and away from others. In the water in which the amoeba live there are usually other organisms, particularly bacteria, on which they feed. When such a bacterium comes in contact with an amoeba, it is taken into its body by becoming enclosed in processes which the amoeba sends out. The enclosed organism then lies in a small clear space in the amoeba, surrounded by fluid which has been shown to differ in its chemical reaction from the general fluid of the interior. This clear space, which may form at any point in the body, corresponds to a stomach in a higher animal and the fluid within it to the digestive fluid or gastric juice. After a time the enclosed organism disappears, it has undergone solution and is assimilated; that is, the substances of which its body was composed have been broken up, the molecules rearranged, and a part has been converted into the substance of the amoeba. If minute insoluble substances, such as particles of carmine, are placed in the water, these may also be taken up by the amoeba; but they undergo no change, and after a time they are cast out. Under the microscope only the gross vital phenomena, motion of the mass, motion within the mass, the reception and disintegration of food particles, and the discharge of inert substances can be observed. The varied and active chemical changes which are taking place cannot be observed.

[Illustration: FIG. 2.--AMOEBA. 1. Nucleus. 2. Contractile vesicle. 3. Nutritive vacuole containing a bacillus.]

Up to the present it has been assumed that the environment of the amoeba is that to which it has become adapted and which is favorable to its existence. Under these conditions its structure conforms to the type of the species, as do also the phenomena which it exhibits, and it can assimilate food, grow and multiply. If, during the observation, a small crystal of salt be placed in the fluid, changes almost instantly take place. Motion ceases, the amoeba appear to shrink into smaller compass, and they become more granular and opaque. If they remain a sufficiently long time in this fluid, they do not regain their usual condition when placed again in fresh water. None of the phenomena which characterized the living amoeba appear: we say they are dead. After a time they begin to disintegrate, and the bacteria contained in the water and on which the amoeba fed now invade their tissue and assist in the disintegration. By varying the duration of the exposure to the salt water or the amount of salt added, a point can be reached where some, but not all, of the amoeba are destroyed. Whether few or many survive depends upon the degree of injury produced. Much the same phenomena can be produced by gradually heating the water in which the amoeba are contained. It is even possible gradually to accustom such small organisms to an environment which would destroy them if suddenly subjected to it, but in the process of adaptation many individuals will have perished.

It is evident from such an experiment that when a living organism is subject to an environment to which it has not become adapted and which is unfavorable, such alterations in its structure may be produced that it is incapable of living even when it is again returned to the conditions natural to it. Such alterations of structure or injuries are called the lesions of disease. We have seen that in certain individuals the injury was sufficient to inhibit for a time only the usual manifestations of life; these returned when the organism was removed from the unfavorable conditions, and with this or preceding it the organisms, if visibly altered, regained the usual form and structure. We may regard this as disease and recovery. In the disease there is both the injury or lesion and the derangement of vital activity dependent upon this. The cause of the disease acted on the organism from without, it was external to it. Whether the injurious external conditions act as in this case by a change in the surrounding osmotic pressure, or by the destruction of ferments within the cell, or by the introduction into the cell of substances which form stable chemical union with certain of its constituents, and thus prevent chemical processes taking place which are necessary for life, the result is the same.

The experiments with the amoeba show also two of the most striking characteristics of living matter. 1. It is adaptable. Under the influence of unusual conditions, alterations in structure and possibly in substance, may take place, in consequence of which the organisms under such external conditions may still exhibit the usual phenomena. The organism cannot adapt itself to such changes without undergoing change in structure, although there may be no evidence of such changes visible. This alteration of structure does not constitute a disease, provided the harmonious relation of the organism with the environment be not impaired. An individual without a liver should not be regarded as diseased, provided there can be such an internal adjustment that all of the vital phenomena could go on in the usual manner without the aid of this useful and frequently maligned organ. 2. It is individual. In the varying degrees of exposure to unfavorable conditions of a more serious nature some, but not all, of the organisms are destroyed; in the slight exposure, few; in the longer, many. Unfavorable conditions which will destroy all individuals of a species exposed to them must be extremely rare.[1] There is no such individuality in non-living things. In a mass of sugar grains each grain shows just the same characteristics and reacts in exactly the same way as all the other grains of the mass. Individuality, however expressed, is due to structural variation. It is almost impossible to conceive in the enormous complexity of living things that any two individuals, whether they be single cells or whether they be formed of cell masses, can be exactly the same. It is not necessary to assume in such individual differences that there be any variation in the amount and character of the component elements, but the individuality may be due to differences in the atomic or molecular arrangements. There are two forms of tartaric-acid crystals of precisely the same chemical formula, one of which reflects polarized light to the left, and the other to the right. All the left-sided crystals and all the right-sided are, however, precisely the same. The number of possible variations in the chemical structure of a substance so complex as is protoplasm is inconceivable.

In no way is the individuality of living matter more strongly expressed than in the resistance to disease. The variation in the degree of resistance to an unfavorable environment is seen in every tale of shipwreck and exposure. In the most extensive epidemics certain individuals are spared; but here care must be exercised in interpreting the immunity, for there must be differences in the degree of exposure to the cause of the epidemic. It would not do to interpret the immunity to bullets in battle as due to any individual peculiarity, save possibly a tendency in certain individuals to remove the body from the vicinity of the bullets; in battle and in epidemics the factors of chance and of prudence enter. No other living organism is so resistant to changes in environment as is man, and to this resistance he owes his supremacy. By means of his intelligence he can change the environment. He is able to resist the action of cold by means of houses, fire and clothing; without such power of intelligent creation of the immediate environment the climatic area in which man could live would be very narrow. Just as disease can be acquired by an unfavorable environment, man can so adjust his environment to an injury that harmony will result in spite of the injury. The environment which is necessary to compensate for an injury may become very narrow. For an individual with a badly working heart more and more restriction of the free life is necessary, until finally the only environment in which life is even tolerably harmonious is between blankets and within the walls of a room.

The various conditions which may act on an organism producing the changes which are necessary for disease are manifold. Lack of resistance to injury, incapacity for adaptation, whether it be due to a congenital defect or to an acquired condition, is not in itself a disease, but the disease is produced by the action on such an individual of external conditions which may be nothing more than those to which the individuals of the species are constantly subject and which produce no harm.

[Illustration: FIG. 3.--A SECTION OF THE SKIN. 1. A hair. Notice there is a deep depression of the surface to form a small bulb from which the hair grows. 2. The superficial or horny layer of the skin; the cells here are joined to form a dense, smooth, compact layer impervious to moisture. 3. The lower layer of cells. In this layer new cells are continually being formed to supply those which as thin scales are cast off from the surface. 4. Section of a small vein. 9. Section of an artery. 8. Section of a lymphatic. The magnification is too low to show the smaller blood vessels. 5. One of the glands alongside of the hair which furnishes an oily secretion. 6. A sweat gland. 7. The fat of the skin. Notice that hair, hair glands and sweat glands are continuous with the surface and represent a downward extension of this. All the tissue below 2 and 3 is the corium from which leather is made.]

[Illustration: FIG. 4.--DIAGRAMMATIC SECTION OF A SURFACE SHOWING THE RELATION OF GLANDS TO THE SURFACE. (_a_) Simple or tubular gland, (_b_) compound or racemose gland.]

All of the causes of disease act on the body from without, and it is important to understand the relations which the body of a highly developed organism such as man has with the world external to him. This relation is effected by means of the various surfaces of the body. On the outside is the skin [Fig. 3], which surface is many times increased by the existence of glands and such appendages to the skin as the hair and nails. A gland, however complicated its structure, is nothing more than an extension of the surface into the tissue beneath [Fig. 4]. In the course of embryonic development all glands are formed by an ingrowth of the surface. The cells which line the gland surface undergo a differentiation in structure which enables them to perform certain definite functions, to take up substances from the same source of supply and transform them. The largest gland on the external surface of the body is the mammary gland [Fig. 5] in which milk is produced; there are two million small, tubular glands, the sweat glands, which produce a watery fluid which serves the purpose of cooling the body by evaporation; there are glands at the openings of the hairs which produce a fatty secretion which lubricates the hair and prevents drying, and many others.

[Illustration: FIG. 5.--A SECTION OF THE MAMMARY GLAND. (_a_) The ducts of the gland, by which the milk secreted by the cells which line all the small openings, is conveyed to the nipple. All these openings are continuous with the surface of the skin. On each side of the large ducts is a vein filled with blood corpuscles.]

[Illustration: FIG. 6.--PHOTOGRAPH OF A SECTION OF THE LUNG OF A MOUSE. x x are the air tubes or bronchi which communicate with all of the small spaces. On the walls of the partitions there is a close network of blood vessels which are separated from the air in the spaces by a thin membrane.]

The external surface passes into the interior of the body forming two surfaces, one of which, the intestinal canal, communicates in two places, at the mouth and anus, with the external surface; and the other, the genito-urinary surface, which communicates with the external surface at one place only. The surface of the intestinal canal is much greater in extent than the surface on the exterior, and finds enormous extensions in the lungs and in the great glands such as the liver and pancreas, which communicate with it by means of their ducts. The extent of surface within the lungs is estimated at ninety-eight square yards, which is due to the extensive infoldings of the surface [Fig 6], just as a large surface of thin cloth can, by folding, be compressed into a small space. The intestinal canal from the mouth to the anus is thirty feet long, the circumference varies greatly, but an average circumference of three inches may safely be assumed, which would give between seven and eight square feet of surface, this being many times multiplied by adding the surfaces of the glands which are connected with it. A diagram of the microscopic structure of the intestinal wall shows how little appreciation of the extent of surface the examination with the naked eye gives [Fig. 7]. By means of the intestinal canal food or substances necessary to provide the energy which the living tissue transforms are introduced. This food is liquefied and so altered by the action of the various fluids formed in the glands of the intestine and poured out on the surface, that it can pass into the interior of the body and become available for the living cells. Various food residues representing either excess of material or material incapable of digestion remain in the intestine, and after undergoing various changes, putrefactive in character, pass from the anus as feces.

By means of the lungs, which represent a part of the surface, the oxygen of the air, which is indispensable for the life of the cells, is taken into the body and carbonic acid removed. The interchange of gases is effected by the blood, which, enclosed in innumerable, small, thin-walled tubes, almost covers the surface, and comes in contact with the air within the lungs, taking from it oxygen and giving to it carbonic acid.

The genito-urinary surface is the smallest of the surfaces. In the male (Fig. 8,--27, 28, 30) this communicates with the general external surface by the small opening at the extremity of the penis, and in the female by the opening into the vagina. In its entirety it consists in a surface of wide extent, comprising in the male the urethra, a long canal which opens into the bladder, and is continuous with ducts that lead into the genital glands or testicles. The internal surface of the bladder is extended by means of two long tubes, the ureters, into the kidneys, and receives the fluid formed in these organs. In the female (Fig 9) there is a shallow external orifice which is continued into the bladder by a short canal, the urethra, the remaining urinary surface being the same as in the male; the external opening also is extended into the short, wide tube of the vagina, which is continuous with the canal of the uterus. This canal is continued on both sides into the Fallopian tubes or oviducts. There is thus in the female a more complete separation of the urinary and the genital surfaces than in the male. Practically all of the waste material of the body which results from cell activity and is passed from the cells into the fluid about them is brought by the blood to the kidneys, and removed by these from the blood, leaving the body as urine.

1. The skull. 2. The brain, showing the convolutions of the gray exterior in which the nerve cells are most numerous. 3. The white matter in the interior of the brain formed of nerve fibres which connect the various parts of this. 4. The small brain or cerebellum. 5. The interior of the nose. Notice the nearness of the upper part of this cavity to the brain. 6. The hard or bony palate forming the roof of the mouth. 7. The soft palate which hangs as a curtain between the mouth and the pharynx. 8. The mouth cavity. 9. The tongue. 10. The beginning of the gullet or oesophagus. 11. The larynx. 12. The windpipe or trachea. 13. The oesophagus. 14. The thyroid gland. 15. The thymus gland or sweetbread. 16. The large vein, vena cava, which conveys the blood from the brain and upper body into the heart. 17-25. Lymph nodes; 17, of the neck; 25, of the abdomen. 18. Cross section of the arch of the aorta or main artery of the body after it leaves the heart. 19. The sternum or breast bone. 20. The cavity of the heart. 21. The liver. 22. The descending aorta at the back of the abdominal cavity. 23. The pancreas. 24. The stomach. 26. Cross section of the intestines. 27. The urinary bladder. 28. The entrance into this of the ureter or canal from the kidney. 29. Cross sections of the pubic bone. 30. The canal of the urethra leading into the bladder. 31. The penis. 32. The spinal cord. 33. The bones composing the spinal column. 34. The sacrum. The space between this and No. 29 is the pelvis. 35. The coccyx or extremity of the back bone. 36. The rectum. 37. The testicles.]

Between these various surfaces is the real interior of the body, in which there are many sorts of living tissues,[2] each, of which, in addition to maintaining itself, has some function necessary for the maintenance of the body as a whole. Many of these tissues have for their main purpose the adjustment and coordination of the activities of the different organs to the needs of the organism as a whole. The activity of certain of the organs is essential for the maintenance of life; without others life can exist for a time only; and others, such as the genital glands, while essential for the preservation of the life of the species, are not essential for the individual. There is a large amount of reciprocity among the tissues; in the case of paired organs the loss of one can be made good by increased activity of the remaining, and certain of the organs are so nearly alike in function that a loss can be compensated for by an increase or modification of the function of a nearly related organ. The various internal parts are connected by means of a close meshwork of interlacing fibrils, the connective tissue, support and strength being given by the various bones. Everywhere enclosing all living cells and penetrating into the densest of the tissues there is fluid. We may even consider the body between the surfaces as a bag filled with fluid into which the various cells and structures are packed.

1. The Fallopian tube which forms the connection between the ovary and the uterus. 2. The ovary. 3. The body of the uterus. 4. The uterine canal. 5. The urinary bladder represented as empty. 6. The entrance of the ureter. 7. The pubic bone. 8. The urethra. 9. The vagina. 10. The common external opening or vulva. 11. The rectum and anus.]

[Illustration: FIG. 10.--THE LUNGS AND WINDPIPE. Parts of the lungs have been removed to show the branching of the air tubes or bronchi which pass into them. All the tubes and the surfaces of the lungs communicate with the inner surface of the body through the larynx.]

The nervous system (Fig. 8) represents one of the most important of the enclosed organs. It serves an important function, not only in regulating and coordinating all functions, but by means of the special senses which are a part of it, the relations of the organism as a whole with the environment are adjusted. It consists of a large central mass, the brain and spinal cord, which is formed in the embryo by an infolding of the external surface, much in the same way that a gland is formed; but the connection with the surface is lost in further development and it becomes completely enclosed. Connected with the central nervous mass, forming really a part of it and developing from it, are the nerves, which appear as white fibrous cords and after dividing and subdividing, are as extremely fine microscopic filaments distributed to all parts of the body. By means of the nerves all impressions are conveyed to the brain and spinal cord; all impulses from this, whether conscious or unconscious, are conveyed to the muscles and other parts. The brain is the sole organ of psychical life; by means of its activity the impressions of the external world conveyed to it through the sense organs are converted into consciousness. Whatever consciousness is, and on this much has been written, it proceeds from or is associated with the activity of the brain cells just as truly as the secretion of gastric juice is due to the activity of the cells of the stomach. The activity of the nervous system is essential for extra-uterine life; life ceases by the cessation of circulation and respiration when either the whole or certain small areas of its tissue are destroyed. In intra-uterine life, with the narrow and unchanging environment of the fluid within the uterine cavity which encloses the foetus, life is compatible with the absence or rudimentary development of the nervous system. The foetus in this condition may be otherwise well developed, and it would be not a misuse of words to say that it was healthy, since it is adjusted to and in harmony with its narrow environment, but it would not be normal. The intra-uterine life of the unborn child, it must be remembered, is carried out by the transmission of energy from the mother to the foetus by means of the close relation between the maternal and foetal circulation. It is only when the free existence demands activities not necessary in intra-uterine life that existence without a central nervous system becomes impossible.

It is essential in so complicated a structure as the body that some apparatus should exist to provide for the interchange of material. The innumerable cell units of the body must have material to provide energy, and useless material which results from their activity must be removed. A household might be almost as much embarrassed by the accumulation of garbage and ashes as by the absence of food and coal. The food, which is taken into the alimentary canal and converted by the digestive fluids into material more directly adapted to the uses of cells, must be conveyed to them. A supply of oxygen is essential for the life of the cells, and the supply which is given by respiration must be carried from the lungs to every cell of the body. All this is effected by the circulation of the blood, which takes place in the system of branching closed tubes in which the blood remains (Fig. 11). Certain of these tubes, the arteries, have strong and elastic walls and serve to convey and distribute the blood to the different organs and tissues. From the ultimate branches of the arteries the blood passes into a close network of tubes, the capillaries, which in enormous numbers are distributed in the tissues and have walls so thin that they allow fluid and gaseous interchange between their contents and the fluid around them to take place. The blood from the capillaries is then collected into a series of tubes, the veins, by which it is returned to the heart. This circulation is maintained by means of a pumping organ or heart, which receives the blood from the veins and by the contraction of its powerful walls forces this into the arteries, the direction of flow being determined as in a pump, by a system of valves. The waste products of cell life pass from the cells into the fluid about them, and are in part directly returned into the blood, but for the greater part pass into it indirectly through another set of vessels, the lymphatics. These are thin-walled tubes which originate in the tissues, and in which there is a constant flow towards the heart, maintained by the constant but varying pressure of the tissue around them, the direction of flow being maintained by numerous valves. The colorless fluid within these vessels is termed "lymph." At intervals along these tubes are small structures termed the lymph nodes, which essentially are filters, and strain out from the fluid substances which might work great injury if they passed into the blood. Between the capillary vessels and the lymphatics is the tissue fluid, in which all the exchange takes place. It is constantly added to by the blood, and returns fluid to the blood and lymph; it gives material to the cells and receives material from them.

[Illustration: FIG. 11.--A DIAGRAMMATIC VIEW OF THE BLOOD VESSELS. An artery (_a_) opens into a system of capillaries, (_c_) and after passing through these collects into a vein (_b_). Notice that the capillaries connect with other vascular territories at numerous points (_d_). If the artery (_a_) became closed the capillaries which it supplies could be filled by blood coming from other sources.]

In addition to the strength and elasticity of the wall of the arteries, which enables them to resist the pressure of the blood, they have the power of varying their calibre by the contraction or expansion of their muscular walls. Many of the organs of the body function discontinuously, periods of activity alternating with comparative repose; during the period of activity a greater blood supply is demanded, and is furnished by relaxation of the muscle fibres which allows the calibre to increase, and with this the blood flow becomes greater in amount. Each part of the body regulates its supply of blood, the regulation being effected by means of nerves which control the tension of the muscle fibres. The circulation may be compared with an irrigation system in which the water supply of each particular field is regulated not by the engineer, but by an automatic device connected with the growing crop and responding to its demands.

[Illustration: FIG. 12.--THE VARIOUS CELLS IN THE BLOOD. (_a_) The red blood cells, single and forming a roll by adhering to one another; (_b_) different forms of the white blood cells; those marked "1" are the most numerous and are phagocytic for bacteria.]

The blood consists of a fluid, the blood plasma, in which numerous cells are contained. The most numerous of these are small cup-shaped cells which contain a substance called _hemoglobin_, to which the red color of the blood is due. There are five million of these cells in a cubic millimeter (a millimeter is .03937 of an inch), giving a total number for the average adult of twenty-five trillion. The surface area of all these, each being one thirty-three hundredth of an inch in diameter, is about thirty-three hundred square yards. The hemoglobin which they contain combines in the lungs with the oxygen in the inspired air, and they give up this indispensable substance to the cells everywhere in the body. There are also eight thousand leucocytes or colorless cells in a cubic millimeter of blood, this giving a total number of four billion in the average adult, and these vary in character and in relative numbers (Fig. 12). The most numerous of these are round and slightly larger than the red cells; they have a nucleus of peculiar shape and contain granules of a definite character. These cells serve an important part in infectious diseases in devouring and destroying parasites. They have power of active independent motion and somewhat resemble certain of the free living unicellular organisms. The blood plasma, when taken from the vessels, clots or passes from a fluid into a gelatinous or semi-solid condition, which is due to the formation within it of a network of fine threads termed fibrin. It is by means of the clotting of the blood that the escape of blood from ruptured vessels is arrested.

Several of the organs of the body, in addition to the formation of secretions which are discharged on the surfaces by means of their ducts, produce also substances which pass directly into the blood or lymph, and have an influence in stimulating or otherwise regulating the activity of other organs. There are also certain organs of glandular structure which are called the _ductless glands_; these are not connected with the surface and all their secretion passes into the blood. It is a part of recent knowledge that the substances produced in these glands are of great importance for the body, some of them even essential for the maintenance of life. In front of the neck is such an organ, the thyroid gland (Fig. 8, 14). Imperfect development or absence of this organ, or an inactive condition of it, produces in the child arrested growth and deficient mental development known as cretinism, and in the adult the same condition gives rise to mental deterioration, swelling of the skin, due to a greater content of water, and loss of hair. This deficiency in the production of thyroid secretion can be made good and the symptoms removed by feeding the patient with similar glands removed from animals. The very complex disease known as exophthalmic goitre, and shown by irregular and rapid action of the heart, protruding eyeballs and a variety of mental symptoms, is also associated with this gland, and occasioned not by a deficiency but by an excess or perversion of its secretion.

Adjoining the thyroid there are four small glands, the parathyroids, each about the size of a split pea. The removal of these glands in animals produces a condition resembling acute poisoning accompanied by spasmodic contraction of the muscles. A small glandular organ at the base of the brain, the pituitary body, produces a secretion, one of the most marked properties of which is a control of growth, particularly that of the bones. Most cases of giantism, combined as they are with imperfect mentality, are due to disease of this gland. There are glands near the kidney which regulate the pressure of the blood in the arteries by causing contraction of their muscular walls. The sexual characteristics in the male and female are due to an internal secretion produced by the respective sexual glands which affects growth, body development and mentality.

So is the body constituted. A series of surfaces, all connected, of enormous size, which enclose a large number of organs and tissues, the activities of which differ, but all are coordinated to serve the purposes of the organism as a whole. We should think of the body not as an assemblage of more or less independent entities, but as a single organism in which all parts are firmly knit together both in structure and in function, as are the components of a single cell.

FOOTNOTES: [1] They do, however, take place, since within comparatively few years whole species have completely disappeared; for example, the great auk and the passenger pigeon. In these cases it is not known what part disease played in the destruction.

[2] A tissue represents an aggregate of similar cells with the intercellular substances in relation with these as connective tissue, muscular tissue, etc. Where such cell aggregates are localized and where the cells are arranged in structures having definite form and size and performing a definite function, it is customary to designate such structures as organs, as the brain, liver, etc.

CHAPTER II

NO SHARP LINE OF DEMARKATION BETWEEN HEALTH AND DISEASE.--THE FUNCTIONAL NUTRITIVE AND FORMATIVE ACTIVITIES OF CELLS.-- DESTRUCTION AND REPAIR CONSTANT PROCESSES IN LIVING MATTER.-- INJURIES TO THE BODY.--THE EFFECT OF HEAT.--THE ACTION OF POISONS.-- THE LESIONS OF DISEASE.--REPAIR.--THE LAWS GOVERNING REPAIR.-- RELATION OF REPAIR TO COMPLEXITY OF STRUCTURE AND AGE.--THE RESERVE FORCE OF THE BODY.-- COMPENSATORY PROCESSES IN THE BODY.-- OLD AGE.--THE DIMINUTION OF RESISTANCE TO THE EFFECT OF THE ENVIRONMENT A PROMINENT FACTOR IN OLD AGE.--DEATH.--HOW BROUGHT ABOUT.--CHANGES IN THE BODY AFTER DEATH.-- THE RECOGNITION OF DEATH.

There is no sharp line separating health from disease; changes in the tissues of the same nature, or closely akin to those which are found in disease, are constantly occurring in a state of health. The importance of parasites in causing disease has led to the conception of disease as almost synonymous with parasitism; but it must be remembered that the presence of parasites living at the expense of the body is perfectly consistent with a state of health. Degeneration, decay and parasitism only become disease factors when the conditions produced by them interfere with the life which is the normal or usual for the individual concerned.

All the changes which take place in the cells are of great importance in conditions of both health and disease, for life consists in coordinated cell activity. The activities of the cells can be divided into those which are nutritive, those which are functional and those which are formative. In the functional activity the cell gives off energy, this loss being made good by the receipt of new energy in the form of nutritive material with which the cell renews itself. In certain cells an exact balance seems to be maintained, but in those cells whose activity is periodic function takes place at the expense of the cell substance, the loss being restored by nutrition during the period of repose. This is shown particularly well in the case of the nerve cells (Fig. 13). Both the functional and nutritive activity can be greatly stimulated, but they must balance; otherwise the condition is that of disease.

[Illustration: FIG 13.--NERVE CELLS OF AN ENGLISH SPARROW (_a_) Cells after a day's full activity, (_b_) cells after a night's repose. In (_a_) the cells and nuclei are shrunken and the smaller clear spaces in the cells are smaller and less evident than in (_b_). (Hodge)]

The formative activity of cells is also essential to the normal state. Destruction of cells is constantly taking place in the body, and more rapidly in certain tissues than in others. Dried and dead cells are constantly and in great numbers thrown off from the surface of the skin: such epidermic appendages as the hair and nails grow and are removed, millions of cells are represented in the beard which is daily removed. Cells are constantly being destroyed on the intestinal surface and in the glands. There is an enormous destruction of the blood cells constantly taking place, certain essential pigments, as that of the bile, being formed from the hemoglobin which the red blood corpuscles contain and which becomes available on their destruction. All such loss of cells must be made good by the formation of new ones and, as in the case of the nutritive and functional activity, the loss and renewal must balance. The formative activity of cells is of great importance, for it is by means of this that wounds heal and diseases are recovered from. This constant destruction and renewal of the body is well known, and it is no doubt this which has given rise to the belief, widely held, that the body renews itself in seven years and that the changes impressed upon it by vaccination endure for this period only. The truth is that the destruction and renewal of most tissues in the body takes place in a much shorter interval, and, as we shall see, this has nothing to do with the changes concerned in vaccination. All these activities of the cells vary in different individuals, in different parts and at different ages.

The lesions or injuries of the body which form so prominent a part of disease vary in kind, degree and situation, depending upon the character of the injurious agent, the duration of its action and the character of the tissue affected. The most obvious injuries are those produced by violence. By a cut, blood vessels are severed, the relations of tissues disturbed, and at the gaping edges of the wound the tissue usually protected by the skin is exposed to the air, resulting in destruction of the cells contained in a thin layer of the surface. The discoloration and swelling of the skin following a blow is due to rupture of vessels and escape of blood and fluid, and further injury may result from the interruption of the circulation.

By the application of heat the tissue may be charred and the albumen of the blood and tissue fluids coagulated. Living cells are very susceptible to the action of heat, a temperature of 130 degrees being the thermal death point, and even lower temperatures are fatal when their action is prolonged. The action of the heat may produce definite coagulation of the fluid within the cells in the same way that the white of an egg is coagulated. Certain of the albumens of the body coagulate at a much lower temperature than the white of the egg (as the myosin, one of the albumens of the muscle which coagulates at 115?F., egg white coagulating at 158?F.), and in addition to such coagulation or without it the ferments within the cell and to the action of which cellular activity is due may be destroyed.

In diseases due to parasites, the parasite produces a change in the tissue in its immediate vicinity often so great as to result in the death of the cells. The most general direct cause of lesions is toxic or poisonous substances, either introduced from without or formed in the body. In the case of the parasitic diseases the mere presence of the parasite in the body produces little or no harm, the injury being caused by poisons which it produces, and which act both locally in the vicinity of the parasite and at a distance, being absorbed and entering the blood stream. How certain of the poisonous substances act is easy to see. Strong caustics act by coagulating the albumen, or by the withdrawal of water from the cell. Other poisons act by forming stable chemical compounds with certain of the cell constituents and thereby preventing the usual chemical processes from taking place. Death from the inhalation of illuminating gas is due to the carbon monoxide contained in this, forming a firm chemical union with the hemoglobin of the red corpuscles so that the function of these as oxygen carriers is stopped.

In order that most poisons may act, it is essential that they enter into the cell, and they cannot do this unless they are able to combine chemically with certain of the cell constituents. To this is due the selective action of many poisons. Morphine, for example, acts chiefly on the cells of the brain; strychnine acts on the cells of the spinal cord which excite motion and thus causes the characteristic muscular spasm. The poisonous substances produced by bacteria, as in the case of diphtheria, act on certain of the organs only. Different animal species owe their immunity to certain poisons to their cells being so constituted that a poison cannot gain entrance into them; pigeons, for example, cannot be poisoned by morphia. Individual variations play an important part also; thus, shellfish are poisonous for certain individuals and not so for others. Owing to the variability of living structures a substance may be poisonous at one time and not at another, as the following example shows. A man, very fond of crab meat, was once violently poisoned after eating crabs, being at that time seemingly in his usual state of health, and no illness resulted in others who had partaken of the same crabs. Two months later a hearty meal of crabs produced no ill result. There are also individuals so constituted that so simple a food as the egg is for them an active poison.

The lesions produced by the action of injurious conditions are usually so distinctive in situation and character that by the examination of the body after death the cause of death can be ascertained. The lesions of diseases may be very obvious to the naked eye, or in other cases only the most careful microscopic examination can detect even the presence of alterations. In the case of poisons the capacity of the cell for adaptation to unusual conditions is of great importance. It is probable that certain changes take place within the cells, owing to which the function can be continued in spite of the unusual conditions which the presence of the poison brings about. It is in this way that the habitual use of such poisons as morphine, alcohol and tobacco, to speak only of those best known, is tolerated. The cell life can become so accustomed to the presence of poisons that the cell activities may suffer in their absence.

Repair of the injuries which the body receives is effected in a variety of ways. We do not know how intracellular repair takes place, but most probably the cells get rid of the injured areas either by ejecting them, or chemical changes are produced in the altered cell substance breaking up and recombining the molecules. When single cells are destroyed, the loss is made good by new formation of cells, the cell loss stimulating the formative activity of the cells in the vicinity. The body maintains a cell and tissue equilibrium, and a loss is in most cases repaired. The blood fluid lost in a hemorrhage is quickly restored by a withdrawal of the fluid from the tissues into the blood, but the cells lost are restored by new formation of cells in the blood-forming organs. The blood cells are all formed in bone marrow and in the lymph nodes, and not from the cells which circulate in the blood, and the stimulus to new cell formation which the loss of blood brings about affects this remote tissue.

In general, repair takes place most easily in tissues of a simple character, and where there is the least differentiation of cell structure for the purposes of function. A high degree of function in which the cell produces material of a complex character necessitates a complex chemical apparatus to carry this out, and a complicated mechanism is formed less easily than a simple one. In certain tissues the cells have become so highly differentiated that all formative activity is lost. Such is the case in the nerve cells of the brain and spinal cord, a loss in which tissue is never repaired by the formation of new cells; and in the muscles the same is true. The least differentiation is seen in those cells which serve the purpose of mechanical protection only, as the cells of the skin, and in these the formative activity is very great. Not only must the usual loss be supplied, but we are all conscious of slight injuries of the surface which are quickly repaired.

Repair, other things being equal, takes place more easily in the young than in the old. New formation of cells goes on with great rapidity in intra-uterine life, the child, beginning its existence as a single cell one two hundred and fiftieth of an inch in diameter, attains in nine months a weight of seven pounds. The only similar rapidity of cell formation is seen in certain tumors; although the body may add a greater amount of weight and in a shorter time, by deposit of fat, this in but slight measure represents a new formation of tissue, but is merely a storage of food material in cells. The remarkable repair and even the new formation of entire parts of the body in the tadpole will not take place in the completely developed frog.

Repair will also take place the more readily the less complicated is the architectural structure of the part affected. When a series of tissues variously and closely related to one another enter into the structure of an organ, there may be new formation of cells; but when the loss involves more than this, the complicated architectural structure will not be completely replaced. A brick which has been knocked out of a building can be easily replaced, but the renewal of an area of the wall is more difficult. In the kidney, for example, the destruction of single cells is quickly made good by new cell formation, but the loss of an area of tissue is never restored. In the liver, on the other hand, which is of much simpler construction, large areas of tissue can be newly formed. For the formation of new cells in a part there must be a sufficient amount of formative material; then the circulation of the blood becomes more active, more blood being brought to the part by dilatation of the vessels supplying it.

Repair after a loss can be perfect or imperfect. The tissue lost can be restored so perfectly that no trace of an injury remains; but when the loss has been extensive, and in a tissue of complex structure, complete restoration does not take place and a less perfect tissue is formed which is called a scar. Examination of the skin in almost anyone will show some such scars which have resulted from wounds. They are also found in the internal organs of the body as the result of injuries which have healed. The scar represents a very imperfect repair. In the skin, for example, the scar tissue never contains such complicated apparatus as hair and sweat glands; the white area is composed of an imperfectly vascularized fibrous tissue which is covered with a modified epidermis. The scar is less resistant than the normal tissue, injury takes place more easily in it and heals with more difficulty.

Loss brought about by the injuries of disease can be compensated for, even when the healing is imperfect, by increased function of similar tissue in the body. There always seems to be in the body under the usual conditions a reserve force, no tissue being worked to its full capacity. Meltzer has compared the reserve force of the body to the factor of safety in mechanical construction. A bridge is constructed to sustain the weight of the usual traffic, but is in addition given strength to meet unusual and unforeseen demands. The stomach provides secretion to meet the usual demands of digestion, but can take care of an unusual amount of food. The work of the heart may be doubled by severe exertions, and it meets this demand by increased force and rapidity of contraction; and the same is true of the muscles attached to the skeleton. The constant exercise of this reserve force breaks down the adjustment. If the weight of the traffic over the bridge be constantly all that it can carry, there quickly comes a time when some slight and unforeseen increase of weight brings disaster. The conditions in the body are rather better than in the case of the bridge, because with the increased demand for activity the heart, for example, becomes larger and stronger, and reserve force rises with the load to be carried, but the ratio of reserve force is diminished.

This discussion of injury and repair leads to the question of old age. Old age, as such, should not be discussed in a book on disease, for it is not a disease; it is just as natural to grow old and to die as it is to be born. Disease, however, differs in many respects in the old as compared with the young and renders some discussion of the condition necessary. Changes are constantly taking place in the body with the advance of years, and in the embryo with the advance of days. In every period of life in the child, in the adult, in the middle-aged and in the old we meet with conditions which were not present at earlier periods. There is no definite period at which the changes which we are accustomed to regard as those of old age begin. This is true of both the external appearances of age and the internal changes. One individual may be fully as old, as far as is indicated by the changes of age, at fifty as another at eighty.

With advancing age certain organs of the body atrophy; they become diminished in size, and the microscopic examination shows absence or diminished numbers of the cells which are peculiar to them. The most striking example of this is seen in the sexual glands of females, and, to a less degree, in those of the male. There is a small mass or glandular tissue at the root of the neck, the thymus, which gradually grows from birth and reaches its greatest size at the age of fifteen, when it begins slowly to atrophy and almost disappears at the age of forty. This is the gland which in the calf is known as the sweetbread and is a delicious and valued article of food. The tonsils, which in the child may be so large as to interfere with breathing and swallowing, have almost disappeared in the adult; and there are other such examples.

In age atrophy is a prominent change. It is seen in the loss of the teeth, in the whitening and loss of the hair, in the thinning of the skin so that it more easily wrinkles, in the thinning and weakening of the muscles so that there is not only diminished force of muscular contraction, but weakening of the muscles of support. The back curves from the action of gravity, the strength of the support of the muscles at the back not counteracting the pull of the weight of the abdominal viscera in front. The bones become more porous and more brittle.

The effect of atrophy is also seen in the diminution of all functions, and in loss of weight in individual organs. That the brain shares in the general atrophy is evident both anatomically and in function. Mental activity is more sluggish, impressions are received with more difficulty, their accuracy may be impaired by accompanying changes in the sense organs, and the concepts formed from the impressions may differ from the usual. The slowness of mental action and the diminution in the range of mental activity excited by impressions, and the slowness of expression, may give a false idea of the value of the judgment expressed. The expression changes, the face becomes more impassive because the facial muscles no longer reflect the constant and ever changing impressions which the youthful sense organs convey to a youthful and active brain. That the young should ape the old, should seek to acquire the gravity of demeanor, to restrain the quick impulse, is not of advantage. Loss of weight of the body as a whole is not so apparent, there being a tendency to fat formation owing to the non-use of fat or fat-forming material which is taken into the body. One of the most evident alterations is a general diminution in the fluid of the tissues, to which is chiefly due the lack of plumpness, the wrinkles of age. The facial appearance of age is given to an infant when, in consequence of a long-continued diarrhoea, the tissues become drained of fluid. Every market-man knows that an old animal is not so available for food, the tissues are tougher, more fibrous, not so easily disintegrated by chewing. This is due to a relative increase in the connective tissue which binds all parts together and is represented in the white fibres of meat.

Senile atrophy is complex in its causes and modes of production. The atrophy affects different organs in different degree and shows great variation in situation, in degree and in progress. Atrophic changes of the blood vessels are of great importance, for this affects the circulation on which the nutrition of all tissues depends. While there is undoubted progressive wear of all tissues, this becomes most evident in the case of the blood vessels of the body. It is rare that arteries which can be regarded as in all respects normal are found in individuals over forty, and these changes progress rapidly with advancing age. So striking and constant are these vascular changes that they seem almost in themselves sufficient to explain the senile changes, and this has been frequently expressed in the remark that age is determined not by years, but by the condition of the arteries. Comparative studies show the falsity of this view, for animals which are but little or not at all subject to arterial disease show senile changes of much the same character as those found in man.

There is another condition which must be considered in a study of causes of age. In the ordinary course of life slight injuries are constantly being received and more or less perfectly repaired. An infection which may but slightly affect the ordinary well-being of the individual may produce a considerable damage. Excess or deficiency or improper food, occasional or continued use of alcohol and other poisons may lead to very definite lesions. Repair after injury is rarely perfect, the repaired tissue is more susceptible to injury, and with advancing age there is constant diminution in the ease and perfection of repair. The effect of the sum of all these changes becomes operative: a vicious circle is established in which injury becomes progressively easier to acquire and repair constantly less perfect. There is some adjustment, however, in that the range of activities is diminished, the environment becomes narrower and the organism adapts its life to that environment which makes the least demands upon it.

Whether there is, entirely apart from all conditions affecting nutrition and the effect of injuries which disturb the usual cell activities, an actual senescence of the cells of the body is uncertain. In the presence of the many factors which influence the obvious diminution of cell activity in the old, it is impossible to say whether the loss of cell activity is intrinsic or extrinsic. The life of the plant cell seems to be immortal; it does not grow old. Trees die owing to accidents or because the tree acquires in the course of its growth a mass of tissue in which there is little or no life, and which becomes the prey of parasites. The growing tissue of a tree is comprised in a thin layer below the bark, and the life of this may seemingly be indefinitely prolonged by placing it in a situation in which it escapes the action of accidental injuries and decay, as by grafting on young trees. Where the nature of the dead wood is such that it is immune from parasites and decay, as in the case of the Sequoias, life seems to be indefinitely prolonged. The growing branches of one of these trees, whose age has been estimated with seeming accuracy at six thousand years, are just as fresh and the tree produces its flowers and fruit in the same degree as a youthful brother of one thousand years. Nor does old age supervene in the unicellular organisms. An amoeba assimilates, grows and multiplies just as long as the environment is favorable.

Old age in itself is seldom a cause of death. In rare cases in the very old a condition is found in which no change is present to which death can be attributed, all organs seem to share alike in the senescence. Death is usually due to some of the accidents of life, a slight infection to which the less resistant body succumbs, or to the rupture of a weakened blood vessel in the brain, or to more advanced decay in some organ whose function is indispensable. The causes and conditions of age have been a fertile source for speculation. Many of the hypotheses have been interesting, that of Metschnikoff, for example, who finds as a dominating influence in causing senescence the absorption of toxic substances formed in the large intestine by certain bacteria. He further finds that the cells of the body which have phagocytic powers turn their activity against cells and tissues which have become weakened. There may be absorption of injurious substances from the intestines which the body in a vigorous condition is able to destroy or to counteract their influence, and these may be more operative in the weaker condition of the body in the old. Phagocytes will remove cells which are dead and often cells which are superfluous in a part, but there is no evidence that this is ever other than a conservative process. Since it is impossible to single out any one condition to which old age is due, the hypothesis of Metschnikoff should have no more regard given it than the many other hypotheses which have been presented.

Death of the body as a whole takes place from the cessation of the action of the central nervous system or of the respiratory system or of the circulation. There are other organs of the body, such as the intestine, kidney, liver, whose function is essential for life, but death does not take place immediately on the cessation of their function. The functions of the heart, the brain and the lungs are intimately associated. Oxygen is indispensable for the life of the tissues, and its supply is dependent upon the integrity of the three organs mentioned, which have been called the tripos of life. Respiration is brought about by the stimulation of certain nerve cells in the brain, the most effective stimulus to these cells being a diminution of oxygen in the blood supplying them. These cells send out impulses to the muscles concerned in inspiration, the chest expands, and air is taken into the lungs. Respiration is then a more complicated process than is the action of the heart, for its contraction, which causes the blood to circulate, is not immediately dependent upon extrinsic influences. Death is usually more immediately due to failure of respiration than to failure of circulation, for the heart often continues beating for a time after respiration has ceased. Thus, in cases of drowning and suffocation, by means of artificial respiration in which air is passively taken into and expelled from the lungs, giving oxygen to the blood, the heart may continue to beat and the circulation continue for hours after all evident signs of life and all sensation has ceased.

By this general death is meant the death of the organism as a whole, but all parts of the body do not die at the same time. The muscles and nerves may react, the heart may be kept beating, and organs of the body when removed and supplied with blood will continue to function. Certain tissues die early, and the first to succumb to the lack of oxygenated blood are the nerve cells of the brain. If respiration and circulation have ceased for as short a time as twelve minutes, life ceases in certain of these cells and cannot be restored. This is again an example of the greater vulnerability of the more highly differentiated structure in which all other forms of cell activity are subordinated to function. There are, however, pretty well authenticated cases of resuscitation after immersion in water for a longer period than twelve minutes, but these cases have not been carefully timed, and time under such conditions may seem longer than it actually is; and there is, moreover, the possibility of a slight gaseous interchange between the blood and the water in the lungs, as in the case of the fish which uses the water for an oxygen supply as the mammal does the air. There are also examples of apparent death or trances which have lasted longer, and the cases of fakirs who have been buried for prolonged periods and again restored to life. In these conditions, however, all the activities of the body are reduced to the utmost, and respiration and circulation, so feeble as to be imperceptible to ordinary observation, suffice to keep the cells living.

With the cessation of life the body is subject to the unmodified action of its physical environment. There is no further production of heat and the body takes the temperature of the surroundings. The only exceptions are rare cases in which such active chemical changes take place in the dead body that heat is generated by chemical action. At a varying interval after death, usually within twelve hours, there is a general contraction and hardening of the muscles due to chemical changes, probably of the nature of coagulation, in them. This begins in the muscles of the head, extends to the extremities, and usually disappears in twenty-four hours. It is always most intense and most rapid in its onset when death is preceded by active muscular exertion. There have been cases of instantaneous death in battle where the body has remained in the position it held at the moment of death, this being due to the instantaneous onset of muscular rigidity. The blood remains fluid for a time after death and settles in the more dependent parts of the body, producing bluish red mottled discolorations. Later the blood coagulates in the vessels. The body loses moisture by evaporation. Drying of the surface takes place where the epidermis is thin, as over the transparent part of the eye and over areas deprived of epidermis. Decomposition and putrefaction of the body due to bacterial action takes place. The bacteria ever present in the alimentary canal make their way from this into the dead tissue. Certain of these bacteria produce gas which accumulates in the tissues and the body often swells enormously. A greenish discoloration appears, which is due to the union of the products of decomposition with the iron in the blood; this is more prominent over the abdomen and appears in lines along the course of the veins. The rapidity with which decomposition takes place varies, and is dependent upon many factors, such as the surrounding temperature, the nutrition of the body at the time of death, the cause of death. It is usually not difficult to recognize that a body is dead. In certain cases, however, the heart's action may be so feeble that no pulse is felt at the wrist, and the current of the expired air may not move a feather held to the nostril or cloud the surface of a mirror by the precipitation of moisture upon it. This condition, combined with unconsciousness and paralysis of all the voluntary muscles, may very closely simulate death. The only absolute evidence of death is given by such changes as loss of body heat, rigor mortis or stiffening of the muscles, coagulation of the blood and decomposition.

CHAPTER III

THE GROWTH OF THE BODY.--GROWTH MORE RAPID IN EMBRYONIC PERIOD.--THE COORDINATION AND REGULATION OF GROWTH.--TUMORS.-- THE GROWTH OF TUMORS COMPARED WITH NORMAL GROWTH.--SIZE, SHAPE AND STRUCTURE OF TUMORS.-- THE GROWTH CAPACITY OF TUMORS

AS SHOWN BY THE INOCULATION OF TUMORS OF MICE.--BENIGN AND MALIGNANT TUMORS.--EFFECT OF INHERITANCE.--ARE TUMORS BECOMING MORE FREQUENT?--THE EFFECT PRODUCED BY A TUMOR ON THE INDIVIDUAL WHO BEARS IT.--RELATION OF TUMORS TO AGE AND SEX.-- THEORIES AS TO THE CAUSE OF TUMORS.--THE PARASITIC THEORY.--THE TRAUMATIC THEORY.--THE EMBRYONIC THEORY.--THE IMPORTANCE OF THE EARLY RECOGNITION AND REMOVAL OF TUMORS.

The power of growth is possessed by every living thing, but growth is not limited to the living. Crystals also will grow, and the rapidity and character of growth and the maximum size of the crystal depends upon the character of the substance which forms the crystal. From the single cell or ovum formed by the union of the male and female sexual cells, growth is continuous until a size corresponding to the type of the species is attained. From this time onward growth is limited to the degree necessary to supply the constant loss of material which the body undergoes. The rapidity of the growth of the body and of its component parts differs at different ages, and becomes progressively less active from its beginning in the ovum until the adult type of the species is attained. As determined by the volume, the embryo increases more than ten thousand times in size during the first month of intra-uterine life. At birth the average weight is six and a half pounds; at the end of the first year eighteen and a half pounds, a gain of twelve pounds; at the end of the second year twenty-three pounds, a gain of four and a half pounds. The growth is coordinated, the size of the single organs bearing a definite ratio, which varies within slight limits, to the size of the body, a large individual having organs of corresponding size. Knowing that the capacity of growth is one of the inherent properties of living matter, it is much easier to understand the continuance of growth than its cessation. It is impossible to avoid the conclusion that there is some internal mechanism of the body which controls and regulates growth. In the first chapter reference was made to organs producing substances which pass directly into the circulation; these substances act by control of the activities of other parts, stimulating or depressing or altering their function. Two of these glands, the thymus, lying in front, where the neck joins the body and which attains its greatest size at puberty, and the pituitary body, placed beneath the brain but forming no part of it, have been shown by recent investigations to have a very definite relation to growth, especially the growth of the skeleton. The growth energy chiefly resides in the skeleton, and if the growing animal has a diet sufficient only to maintain the body weight, the skeleton will continue to grow at the expense of the other tissues, literally living upon the rest of the body. Disease of the glands mentioned leading to an increase or diminution or alteration of their function may not only inhibit or unduly increase the growth of the skeleton, but may also interfere with the sexual development which accompanies the skeleton growth.

The difficulties which arise in an endeavor to comprehend normal growth are greater when the growth of tumors is considered. A tumor is a mass of newly formed tissue which in structure, in growth, and the relations which it forms with adjoining tissues departs to a greater or less degree from the type of the tissue to which it is related in structure or from which it originates. It is an independent structure which, like a parasite, grows at the expense of the body, contributing nothing to it, and its capacity for growth is unlimited. A tumor cannot be considered as an organ, its activities not being coordinated with those of the body. A part of the body it certainly is, but in the household economy it is to be considered as a wild and lawless guest, not influenced by or conforming with the regulations of the household. The rapidity of growth varies; certain tumors for years increase but little in size, while others may be seen to increase from day to day. The growth is often intermittent, periods of great activity of growth alternating with periods of quiescence. The nutrition and growth of a tumor is only slightly influenced by the condition of nutrition of the bearer. Its cells have a greater avidity for food than have those of the body, and, like the growing bones of an insufficiently fed animal, growth in some cases seems to take place at the expense of the body, the normal cells not obtaining sufficient nutriment to repair their waste.

A tumor may be of any size: so small as to be invisible to the naked eye, or its weight may exceed that of the individual who bears it. The limitations to its growth are extrinsic and not intrinsic. There is no distinct color. Certain tumors have color which depends upon the presence of a dark brown or black pigment within the cells. H 鎚 orrhages within them are not infrequent, and they may be colored by the blood or by pigments formed from it. Usually they have a gray color modified by their varying vascularity, or the cut surface may be mottled due to areas of cell degeneration. The consistency varies; some tumors are so soft that they can be pressed through a sieve, others are of stony hardness. There is no distinct shape, this being influenced by the nature of the tumor, the manner of growth and situation. When the tumor grows on or near a surface, it may project from this and be attached by a narrow band only; in the interior of the body it may be irregular in outline, round or lobular, the shape being influenced by many factors. Tumors like the tissues of the normal body are nourished by the blood and contain blood vessels often in great numbers.

A tumor arises by the cells of a part of the body beginning to grow and taking on the characteristics of a tumor. Its growth is independent, the cells of the adjoining tissue taking no part in it. The tissue in the vicinity of the tumor is partly pushed aside by the mass, or the tumor grows into it and the tissue disappears as the tumor advances. The destruction of the surrounding tissue is brought about partly by the pressure which the tumor exerts, partly by the compression of the blood vessels or the blood supply of the organs is diverted to the tumor.

The characteristics of a tumor are due to the cells which it contains (Fig 14). These often become separated from the main mass and are carried by the blood into other parts of the body, where they grow and form tumors similar in character to the parent tumor. In the extraordinary capacity for growth possessed by tumor cells, they resemble vegetable rather than animal cells. There is no limit to the growth of a tumor save by the death of the individual who bears it, thus cutting off the supply of nutrition. The cells of tumors peculiar to man show a narrow range of adaptation. They will grow only in the body of the individual to whom the tumor belongs, and die when grafted on another individual. In the case of tumors which arise in animals, pieces of the tumor when grafted on another animal of the same species will grow, and in this way the growth capacity of the tumor cells has been estimated. Thus, by transplanting a small section of a mouse tumor into other mice, the small transplanted fragments will in two weeks grow to the size of filberts, and each of these will furnish material to engraft upon ten mice. These new tumors are similar in character to the original tumor, and really represent parts of it in the same way that all the Baldwin apples in the world are parts of the original tree which was found in Baldwinville many years ago, and as all the Concord grape vines are really parts of the original vine. It has been estimated that if all the growth capacity of this mouse tumor were availed of by the successive inoculation of other mice, a mass of tumor several times the diameter of the sun would grow in two years. The condition of the individual seems to exert no influence upon the growth of the tumor. Growth may be as rapid when the bearer is in a condition of extreme emaciation as it is when the bearer is well nourished and robust.

[Illustration: FIG 14.--PHOTOGRAPH OF A MICROSCOPIC PREPARATION FROM A CANCER OF THE UTERUS. A large mass of cells is extending into the tissue of the uterus which is shown as the fibrous structure. Such a cell mass penetrating into the tissue represents the real cancer, the tissue about the cell masses bear the blood vessels which nourish the tumor cells.]

Those tumors which grow rapidly and invade and destroy the surrounding tissue are called malignant tumors or cancers, but in a strict sense no tumor can be regarded as benign, for none can serve a useful purpose. A tumor after a period of slow growth can begin to grow rapidly. Tumors may arise in any part of the body, but there are certain places of preference particularly for the more malignant tumors. These are places where the cells naturally have a marked power of growth, and especially where growth is intermittent as in the uterus and mammary gland.

Little is known in regard to the influence of inheritance on the formation of tumors. Study of the tumors of mice show a slightly greater susceptibility to tumor formation in the progeny of mice who have developed tumors. Studies of human families seem to show that heredity has a slight influence, but in the frequency of tumors such statistical evidence is of little value. The question of inheritance has much bearing on the origin of tumors. If the tumor is accidental and due entirely to extraneous causes, inheritance is not probable; but if there is some predisposition to tumor formation in certain individuals due to some peculiarity, then inheritance may exert an influence.

The question as to whether tumors are an increasing cause of disease is equally difficult of solution. The mortality statistics, if taken at their face value, show an enormous increase in frequency; but there are many factors which must be considered and which render the decision difficult and doubtful. Tumors are largely a prerogative of age, and the increased duration of life which preventive medicine has brought about brings more people into the age when tumors are more common. Owing to the greater skill in the diagnosis of tumors, especially those of the internal organs, they are now recognized more frequently and more deaths are correctly ascribed to them. Deaths from tumors were formerly often purposely concealed and attributed to some other cause.

No age is immune to tumors. They may be present at birth or develop shortly afterwards. The age from five to twenty years is the most free from them, that from forty-five to sixty-five the most susceptible, particularly to the more malignant forms.

A tumor is a local disease. The growing tissue of the tumor is the disease, and it is evident that if the entire tumor were removed the disease would be cured. This is the end sought by surgical interference, but notwithstanding seemingly thorough removal, the tumor often reappears after an interval of months or years. There are many conditions which may render the complete removal of a tumor difficult or impossible. It is often impossible to ascertain just how far the tumor cells have invaded the neighboring structures; the situation of the tumor may be such that an extended removal would injure organs which are essential for life, or at the time of removal the tumor cells may have been conveyed elsewhere by the blood or lymphatic vessels.

Successful removal depends mainly upon the length of time the tumor has been growing. At an early stage even the most malignant tumor may be successfully removed. It is evident from this how disastrous may be the neglect of proper surgical treatment of a tumor. The time may be very short between the first evidence of the presence of a tumor and the development of a condition which would render complete removal impossible.

The effect of a tumor upon its bearer depends upon its character and situation. Pain is very commonly present, and is due to the pressure which the growing tumor exerts upon the sensory nerves. Pain may, however, not be present or appear only at the last. A condition of malnutrition and emaciation often results due to the passage into the blood of injurious substances formed in the tumor, or to the destruction of important organs by the growing tumor. The growth of a tumor in the intestine may obstruct or close the canal and thus interfere with nutrition.

The cause or causes of tumors are unknown. We know that the tumor represents essentially an abnormal growth, and that this growth is due to new formation of cells. In certain cases the tumor repeats the structure of the organ or tissue in which it originates, in others it departs widely from this;

always, however, its structure resembles structures found in the body at some period of life. The tumor cells, like all other cells of the body, grow by means of the nutriment which the body supplies; they have no intrinsic sources of energy. The great problem is what starts the cells to grow and why the growth differs from that of normal tissue, why it is not regulated and coordinated as are other forms of growth. When a small piece of the skin, for instance, is cut out growth as rapid as that in tumors takes place in the adjoining cells, but it ceases when the loss is restored. The same is true when a piece of the liver is removed.

Various hypotheses have been formed to explain the tumor, all of them of interest, and they have had great importance in that the attempt to prove or disprove the hypothesis by continued observation and experiment along definite lines has produced new knowledge. The various theories as to cause may be divided into three heads.

The parasitic theory. This supposes that a living parasite invades the body, and by its presence excites the cells of certain tissues to grow in tumor form. It is known that active growth of the cells of the body can be excited in a number of ways, by chemical substances such as certain of the coal tar products, and that it often takes place under the influence of bacteria. It is further known that parasites can produce tumor-like growths in plants. The large, rough excrescences on the oaks are produced by a fly which lays its eggs in or beneath the bark, and the larva which develops from the egg secretes a substance which causes the cells about it to multiply, and a huge mass is formed which serves the developing insect for both food and protection. Large tumor-like masses are formed on the roots and stalk of cabbages as the result of the invasion of the cells by a minute organism: the tumors of olive trees are due to a bacterium; the peculiar growths on cedar trees, the so-called "witches' brooms," are produced by a fungus, and there are many other such examples. These have many analogies with tumors in animals. Under the stimulus of the parasite the cells seem to have unlimited growth capacity and a greater nutritive avidity than have the normal plant cells; the character of the mass produced differs as does the tumor, to a greater or less extent, from the normal growth; on the cedar, for instance, the "witches' broom" consists of a thick mass of foliage with small stems less green than the usual foliage, the leaves wider and not so closely applied to the stems. The entire plant suffers in its nutrition and a condition resembling tumor cachexia[1] is produced, and there are no fundamental differences between the plant and animal tumors. Support has also been given to the parasitic theory by the discovery within tumor cells of bodies which were supposed to be a peculiar sort of parasite. If the truth of the parasitic theory could be proved, there would be justifiable expectation that the tumor disease might be controlled as are many of the parasitic diseases, but the hypothesis awaits the demonstration of its correctness. Despite the study of tumors which is being actively pursued in many places and by the most skilled investigators, no parasites have been found in animal tumors; the objects previously described as parasites have been found not to be such. It is difficult to bring in accord with the parasitic theory the great variation in tumor structure, the relation of certain tumors, as the malignant tumors of the breast and uterus, with the age of the bearer, the congenital tumors which develop in intra-uterine life, and there are many other conditions which oppose the theory.

The traumatic[2] theory. There is much in favor of this. In a certain number of cases tumors do develop at the site of injuries. The coincidence of injury and tumor is apt to be overestimated because of the strong tendency to connect succeeding events. Tumors are not most common on those parts of the body which are most exposed to injury. They are rare, for instance, on the hands and feet, and very rarely do they appear at the site of wounds caused by surgical operations. For those tumors which develop in intra-uterine life it is difficult to assign injury as a cause. There does, however, seem to be a relation between tumors and injuries of a certain character. The natives of Cashmere use in winter for purposes of heat a small charcoal stove which they bind on the front of the body; burns often result and tumors not infrequently develop at the site of such burns. Injuries of tissue which are produced by the X-ray not infrequently result in tumor formation and years may elapse between the receipt of the injury and the development of the tumor. These X-ray injuries are of a peculiar character, their nature but imperfectly understood, and the injured tissues seem to have lost the capacity for perfect repair.

In regard to the possible action of both injuries and parasites in causing tumors, the possibility that their effects on different individuals may not be the same must be considered. In addition to the trauma or the parasite which may be considered as extrinsic factors, there may be conditions of the body, intrinsic factors, which favor their action in tumor development. The peculiar tissue growth within the uterus called decidua, which occurs normally in pregnancy and serves to fasten the developing ovum to the inner lining of the uterus, may be produced experimentally. This growth depends upon two factors, an internal secretion derived from the ovary and the introduction into the uterus of a foreign body of some sort; in the case of pregnancy the developing embryo acts as the foreign body. It is not impossible that some variation in the complex relations which determine normal growth may be one factor, possibly the most important, in tumor formation.

Another theory is that the tumor is the result of imperfect embryonic development. The development of the child from the ovum is the result of a continued formation and differentiation of cells. A cell mass is first produced, and the cells in this differentiate into three layers called ectoderm, entoderm and mesoderm, from which the external and internal surfaces and the enclosed tissues respectively develop, and the different organs are produced by growth of the cells of certain areas of these layers. The embryonic theory assumes that in the course of embryonic development not all the cell material destined for the formation of individual organs is used up for this purpose, that certain of the embryonic cells become enclosed in the developing organs, they retain the embryonic capacity for growth and tumors arise from them. There is no doubt that something like this does take place. There is a relation between malformations due to imperfect development of the embryo and tumors, the two conditions occurring together too frequently to be regarded as mere coincidence. Also tumors may occur in parts of the body in which there is no tissue capable of forming structures which may be present in the tumors. The theory, however, is not adequate, but it may be among the factors.

The problems concerned in the nature and cause of tumors are the most important in medicine at the present time. No other form of disease causes a similar amount of suffering and anxiety, which often extends over years and makes a terrible drain on the sympathy and resources of the family. The only efficient treatment for tumors at the present time is removal by surgical operation, and the success of the operation is in direct ratio to the age of the tumor, the time which elapses from its beginning development. It is of the utmost importance that this should be generally recognized, and the facts relating to tumors become general knowledge. Tumors form one of the most common causes of death (after the age of thirty-five one in every ten individuals dies of tumor); medical and surgical resources are, in many cases, powerless to afford relief and the tumor stands as a bar to the attainment of the utopia represented by a happy and comfortable old age, and a quiet passing. Every possible resource should be placed at the disposal of the scientific investigation of the subject, for with knowledge will come power to relieve.

FOOTNOTES: [1] By cachexia is understood a condition of malnutrition and emaciation which is usually accompanied by a pale sallow color of the skin.

[2] By trauma is understood a wound or injury of any sort.

CHAPTER IV

THE REACTIONS OF THE TISSUES OF THE BODY TO INJURIES.-- INFLAMMATION.-- THE CHANGES IN THE BLOOD IN THIS.--THE EMIGRATION OF THE CORPUSCLES OF THE BLOOD.--THE EVIDENT CHANGES IN THE INJURED PART AND THE MANNER IN WHICH THESE ARE PRODUCED.--HEAT, REDNESS, SWELLING AND PAIN.--THE PRODUCTION OF BLISTERS BY SUNBURN.--THE CHANGES IN THE CELLS OF AN INJURED PART.--THE CELLS WHICH MIGRATE FROM THE BLOOD-VESSELS ACT AS PHAGOCYTES.--THE MACROPHAGES.--THE MICROPHAGES.--CHEMOTROPISM.--THE HEALING OF INFLAMMATION.--THE REMOVAL OF THE CAUSE.--CELL REPAIR AND NEW FORMATION.--NEW FORMATION OF BLOOD-VESSELS.--ACUTE AND CHRONIC INFLAMMATION.--THE APPARENTLY PURPOSEFUL CHARACTER OF THE CHANGES IN INFLAMMATION.

Injury and repair have already been briefly considered in their relation to the normal body and to old age; there are, however, certain phenomena included under the term inflammation which follow the more extensive injuries and demand a closer consideration than was given in Chapter II.

These phenomena differ in degree and character; they are affected by the nature of the injurious agent and the intensity of its action, by the character of the tissue which is affected and by variations in individual resistance to injury. A blow which would have no effect upon the general surface of the body may produce serious results if it fall upon the eye, and less serious results for a robust than for a weak individual.

Most of the changes which take place after an injury and their sequence can be followed under the microscope. If the thin membrane between the toes of a living frog be placed under the microscope the blood vessels and the circulating blood can be distinctly seen in the thin tissue between the transparent surfaces. The arteries, the capillaries and veins can be distinguished, the arteries by the changing rapidity of the blood stream within them, there being a quickening of the flow corresponding with each contraction of the heart; the veins appear as large vessels in which the blood flows regularly (Fig. 11). Between the veins and arteries is a large number of capillaries with thin transparent walls and a diameter no greater than that of the single blood corpuscles; they receive the blood from the arteries and the flow in them is continuous. The white and red blood corpuscles can be distinguished, the red appearing as oval discs and the white as colorless spheres. In the arteries and veins the red corpuscles remain in the centre of the vessels appearing as a rapidly moving red core, and between this core and the wall of the vessels is a layer of clear fluid in which the white corpuscles move more slowly, often turning over and over as a ball rolls along the table.

If, now, the web be injured by pricking it or placing some irritating substance upon it, a change takes place in the circulation. The arteries and the veins become dilated and the flow of blood more rapid, so rapid, indeed, that it is difficult to distinguish the single corpuscles. In a short while the rapidity of flow in the dilated vessels diminishes, becoming slower than the normal, and the separation between the red and white corpuscles is not so evident. In the slowly moving stream the white corpuscles move much more slowly than do the red, and hence accumulate in the vessels lining the inner surface and later become attached to this and cease to move forward. The attached corpuscles then begin to move as does an amoeba, sending out projections, some one of which penetrates the wall, and following this the corpuscles creep through. Red corpuscles also pass out of the vessels, this taking place in the capillaries; the white corpuscles, on the other hand, pass through the small veins. Not only do the white corpuscles pass through the vessels, but the blood fluid also passes out. The corpuscles which have passed into the tissue around the vessels are carried away by the outstreaming fluid, and the web becomes swollen from the increased amount of fluid which it contains. The injured area of the web is more sensitive than a corresponding uninjured area and the foot is more quickly moved if it be touched. If the injury has been very slight, observation of the area on the following day will show no change beyond a slight dilatation of the vessels and a great accumulation of cells in the tissue.

Everyone has experienced the effect of such changes as have been described in this simple experiment. An inflamed part on the surface of the body is redder than the normal, swollen, hot and painful. The usual red tinge of the skin is due to the red blood contained in the vessels, and the color is intensified when, owing to the dilatation, the vessels contain more blood. The inflamed area feels hot, and if the temperature be taken it may be two or three degrees warmer than a corresponding area. The increased heat is due to the richer circulation. Heat is produced in the interior of the body chiefly in the muscles and great glands, and the increased afflux of blood brings more heat to the surface. A certain degree of swelling of the tissue is due to the dilatation of the vessels; but this is a negligible factor as compared with the effect of the presence of the fluid and cells of the exudate.[1] The fluid distends the tissue spaces, and it may pass from the tissue and accumulate on surfaces or in the large cavities within the body. The greatly increased discharge from the nose in a "cold in the head" is due to the exudation formed in the acutely inflamed tissue, and which readily passes through the thin epithelial covering. Various degrees of inflammation of the skin may be produced by the action of the sun, the injury being due not to the heat but to the actinic rays. In a mild degree of exposure only redness and a strong sense of heat are produced, but in prolonged exposure an exudate is formed which causes the skin to swell and blisters to form, these being due to the exudate which passes through the lower layers of the cells of the epidermis and collects beneath the impervious upper layer, detaching this from its connections. If a small wad of cotton, soaked in strong ammonia, be placed on the skin and covered with a thimble and removed after two minutes, minute blisters of exudate slowly form at the spot.

The pain in an inflamed part is due to a number of factors, but chiefly to the increased pressure upon the sensory nerves caused by the exudate. The pain varies so greatly in degree and character that parts which ordinarily have little sensation may become exquisitely painful when inflamed. The pain is usually greater when the affected part is dense and unyielding, as the membranes around bones and teeth. The pain is often intermittent, there being acute paroxysms synchronous with the pulse, this being due to momentary increase of pressure when more blood is forced into the part at each contraction of the heart. The pain may also be due to the direct action of an injurious substance upon the sensory nerves, as in the case of the sting of an insect where the pain is immediate and most intense before the exudate has begun to appear.

When an inflamed area is examined, after twenty-four hours, by hardening the tissue in some of the fluids used for this purpose and cutting it into very thin slices by means of an instrument called a microtome, the microscope shows a series of changes which were not apparent on naked eye examination. The texture is looser, due to the exudate which has dilated all the spaces in the tissue. Red and white corpuscles in varying numbers and proportions infiltrate the tissue; all the cells which belong to the part, even those forming the walls of the vessels, are swollen, the nuclei contain more chromatin, and the changes in the nuclei which indicate that the cells are multiplying appear. The blood vessels are dilated, and the part in every way gives the indication of a more active life within it. There are also evidences of the tissue injury which has called forth all the changes which we have considered. (Fig. 15.)

[Illustration: FIG. 15--A SECTION OF AN INFLAMED LUNG SHOWING THE EXUDATE WITHIN THE AIR SPACES. Compare this with Fig 6. Fig 15 is from the human lung, in which the air spaces are much larger than in the mouse.]

The microscopic examination of any normal tissue of the body shows within it a variable number of cells which have no intimate association with the structure of the part and do not seem to participate in its function. They are found in situations which indicate that these cells have power of active independent motion. In the inflamed tissue a greatly increased number of these cells is found, but they do not appear until the height of the process has passed, usually not before thirty-six or forty-eight hours after the injury has been received. The numbers present depend much upon the character of the agent which has produced the injury, and they may be more numerous than the ordinary leucocytes which migrate from the blood vessels.

All these changes which an injured part undergoes are found when closely analyzed to be purposeful; that is, they are in accord with the conditions under which the living matter acts, and they seem to facilitate the operation of these conditions. It has been said that the life of the organism depends upon the coordinated activity of the living units or cells of which it is composed. The cells receive from the blood material for the purpose of function, for cell repair and renewal, and the products of waste must be removed. In the injury which has been produced in the tissue all the cells have suffered, some possibly displaced from their connections, others may have been completely destroyed, others have sustained varying degrees of injury. If the injury be of an infectious character, that is, produced by bacteria, these may be present in the part and continue to exert injury by the poisonous substances which they produce, or if the injury has been produced by the action of some other sort of poison, this may be present in concentrated form, or the injury may have been the result of the presence of a foreign body in the part. Under these conditions, since the usual activities of the cells in the injured part will not suffice to restore the integrity of the tissue, repair and cell formation must be more active than usual, any injurious substances must be removed or such changes must take place in the tissue that the cell life adapts itself to new conditions.

[Illustration: FIG. 16.--PHAGOCYTOSIS. a, b, c are the microphages or the bacterial phagocytes. (_a_) Contains a number of round bacteria, and (_b_) similar bacteria arranged in chains, and (_c_) a number of rod-shaped bacteria (_d_) Is a cell phagocyte or macrophage which contains five red blood corpuscles.]

All life in the tissues depends upon the circulation of the blood. There is definite relation between the activity of cells and the blood supply; a part, for instance, which is in active function receives a greater supply of blood by means of dilatation of the arteries which supply it. If the body be exactly balanced longitudinally on a platform, reading or any exercise of the brain causes the head end to sink owing to the relatively greater amount of blood which the brain receives when in active function. The regulation of the blood supply is effected by means of nerves which act upon the muscular walls of the arteries causing, by the contraction or the relaxation of the muscle, diminution or dilatation of the calibre of the vessel. After injury the dilatation of the vessels with the greater afflux of blood to the part is the effect of the greatly increased cell activity, and is a necessity for this. In many forms of disease it has been found that by increasing the blood flow to a part and producing an active circulation in it, that recovery more readily takes place and many of the procedures which have been found useful in inflammation, such as hot applications, act by increasing the blood flow. So intimate is the association between cell activity, as shown in repair and new formation of cells, and the blood flow, that new blood vessels frequently develop by means of which the capacity for nutrition is still more increased. The cornea or transparent part of the eye contains no blood vessels, the cells which it contains being nourished by the tissue fluid which comes from the outside and circulates in small communicating spaces. If the centre of the cornea be injured, the cells of the blood vessels in the tissue around the cornea multiply and form new vessels which grow into the cornea and appear as a pink fringe around the periphery; when repair has taken place the newly formed vessels disappear.

The exudate from the blood vessels in various ways assists in repair. An injurious substance in the tissue may be so diluted by the fluid that its action is minimized. A small crystal of salt is irritating to the eye, but a much greater amount of the same substance in dilute solution causes no irritation. The poisonous substances produced by bacteria are diluted and washed away from the part by the exudate. Not only is there a greater amount of tissue fluid in the inflamed part, but the circulation of this is also increased, as is shown by comparing the outflow in the lymphatic vessels with the normal. The fluid exudate which has come from the blood and differs but slightly from the blood fluid exerts not only the purely physical action of removing and diluting injurious substances, but in many cases has a remarkable power, exercised particularly on bacterial poisons, of neutralizing poisons or so changing their character that they cease to be injurious.

We have learned, chiefly from the work of Metschnikoff, that those white corpuscles or leucocytes which migrate from the vessels in the greatest numbers have marked phagocytic properties, that is, they can devour other living things and thus destroy them just as do the amoeb? In inflammations produced by bacteria there is a very active migration of these cells from the vessels; they accumulate in the tissue and devour the bacteria. They may be present in such masses as to form a dense wall around the bacteria, thus acting as a physical bar to their further extension. The other form of amoeboid cell, which Metschnikoff calls the macrophage, has more feeble phagocytic action towards bacteria, and these are rarely found enclosed within them. It is chiefly by means of their activity that other sorts of substances are removed. They often contain dead cells or cell fragments, and when hemorrhage takes place in a tissue they enclose and remove the granules of blood pigment which result. They often join together, forming connected masses, and surround such a foreign body as a hair, or a thread which the surgeon places in a wound to close it. They may destroy living cells, and do this seemingly when certain cells are in too great numbers and superfluous in a part, their action tending to restore the cell equilibrium. The foreign cells do even more than this: they themselves may be devoured by the growing cells of the tissue, seemingly being actuated by the same supreme idea of sacrifice which led Buddha to give himself to the tigress.

The explanation of most of the changes which take place in inflammation is obvious. It is a definite property of all living things that repair takes place after injury, and certain of the changes are only an accentuation of those which take place in the usual life; but others, such as the formation of the exudate, are unusual; not only is the outpouring of fluid greatly increased, but its character is changed. In the normal transudation[2] the substances on which the coagulation of the blood depends pass through the vessel wall to a very slight extent, but the exudate may contain the coagulable material in such amounts that it easily clots. The interchange between the fluid outside the vessels and the blood fluid takes place by means of filtration and osmosis. There is a greater pressure in the vessels than in the fluid outside of them, and the fluid filters through the wall as fluid filters through a thin membrane outside of the body. Osmosis takes place when two fluids of different osmotic pressure are separated by animal membrane. Difference in osmotic pressure is due to differences in molecular concentration, the greater the number of molecules the greater is the pressure, and the greater rapidity of flow is from the fluid of less pressure to the fluid of greater pressure. The molecular concentration of tissue and blood fluid is constantly being equalized by the process of osmosis. In the injured tissue the conditions are more favorable for the fluid of the blood to pass from the vessels: by filtration, because owing to the dilatation of the arteries there is increased amount of blood and greater pressure within the vessels, and the filtering membrane is also thinner because the same amount of membrane (here the wall of the vessel) must cover the larger surface produced by the dilatation. It is, moreover, very generally believed that there are minute openings in the walls of the capillaries, and these would become larger in the dilated vessel just as openings in a sheet of rubber become larger when this is stretched. Osmosis towards the tissue is favored because, owing to destructive processes the molecular pressure in the injured area is increased; an injured tissue has been shown to take up fluid more readily outside of the body than a corresponding uninjured tissue. The slowing of the blood stream, in spite of the dilatation of the vessels, is due to the greater friction of the suspended corpuscles on the walls of the vessels. This is due to the loss from the blood of the outstreaming fluid and the relative increase in the number of corpuscles, added to by the unevenness of surface which the attached corpuscles produce.

The wonderful migration of the leucocytes, which seems to show a conscious protective action on their part, takes place under the action of conditions which influence the movement of cells. When an actively moving amoeba is observed it is seen that the motion is not the result of chance, for it is influenced by conditions external to the organism; certain substances are found to attract the amoebae towards them and other substances to repel them. These influences or forces affecting the movements of organisms are known as tropisms, and play a large part in nature; the attraction of various organisms towards a source of light is known as heliotropism, and there are many other instances of such attraction. The leucocytes as free moving cells also come under the influence of such tropisms. When a small capillary tube having one end sealed is partially filled with the bacteria which produce abscess and placed beneath the skin it quickly becomes filled with leucocytes, these being attracted by the bacteria it contains. Dead cells exert a similar attraction for the large phagocytes. Such attraction is called chemotropism and is supposed to be due in the cases mentioned, to the action of chemical substances such as are given off by the bacteria or the dead cells. The direction of motion is due to stimulation of that part of the body of the leucocyte which is towards the source of the stimulus. The presence in the injured part of bacteria or of injured and dead cells exerts an attraction for the leucocytes within the vessels causing their migration. When the centre of the cornea is injured, this tissue having no vessels, all the vascular phenomena take place in the white part of the eye immediately around the cornea, this becoming red and congested. The migration of leucocytes from the vessels takes place chiefly on the side towards the cornea, and the migrated cells make their way along the devious tracts of the communicating lymph spaces to the area of injury. The objection may be raised that it is difficult to think of a chemical substance produced in an injured area no larger than a millimeter, diffusing through the cornea and reaching the vessels outside this in such quantity and concentration as to affect their contents, nor has there been any evidence presented that definite chemical substances are produced in injured tissues; but there is no difficulty in view of the possibilities. It is not necessary to assume that an actual substance so diffuses itself, but the influence exerted may be thought of as a force, possibly some form of molecular motion, which is set in action at the area of injury and extends from this. No actual substance passes along a nerve when it conveys an impulse.

We have left the injured area with an increased amount of fluid and cells within it, with the blood vessels dilated and with both cells and fluid streaming through their walls, and the cells belonging to the area actively repairing damages and multiplying. The process will continue as long as the cause which produces the injury continues to act, and will gradually cease with the discontinuance of this action, and this may be brought about in various ways. A foreign body may be mechanically removed, as when a thorn is plucked out; or bacteria may be destroyed by the leucocytes; or a poison, such as the sting of an insect, may be diluted by the exudate until it be no longer injurious, or it may be neutralized. Even without the removal of the cause the power of adaptation will enable the life of the affected part to go on, less perfectly perhaps, in the new environment. The excess of fluid is removed by the outflow exceeding the inflow, or it may pass to some one of the surfaces of the body, or in other cases an incision favors its escape. The excess of cells is in part removed with the fluid, in part they disappear by undergoing solution and in part they are devoured by other cells. With the diminishing cell activity the blood vessels resume their usual calibre, and when the newly formed vessels become redundant they disappear by undergoing atrophy in the same way as other tissues which have become useless.

When these changes take place rapidly the inflammation is said to be acute, and chronic when they take place slowly. Chronic inflammation is more complex than is the acute, and there is more variation in the single conditions. The chronicity may be due to a number of conditions, as the persistence of a cause, or to incompleteness of repair which renders the part once affected more vulnerable, to such a degree even that the ordinary conditions to which it is subjected become injurious. A chronic inflammation may be little more than an almost continuous series of acute inflammations, with repair continuously less perfect. Chronic imflammations are a prerogative of the old as compared with the young, of the weak rather than the strong.

FOOTNOTES: [1] The term exudation is used to designate the passing of cells and fluid from the vessels in inflammation; the material is the exudate.

[2] By transudation is meant the constant interchange between the blood and the tissue fluid.

CHAPTER V

INFECTIOUS DISEASES.--THE HISTORICAL IMPORTANCE OF EPIDEMICS OF DISEASE.--THE LOSSES IN BATTLE CONTRASTED WITH THE LOSSES IN ARMIES PRODUCED BY--INFECTIOUS DISEASES.--THE DEVELOPMENT OF KNOWLEDGE OF EPIDEMICS.--THE VIEWS OF HIPPOCRATES AND ARISTOTLE.--SPORADIC AND EPIDEMIC DISEASES.--THE THEORY OF THE EPIDEMIC CONSTITUTION.--THEORY THAT THE CONTAGIOUS MATERIAL IS LIVING.--THE DISCOVERY OF BACTERIA BY LOEWENHOECK IN 1675.--THE RELATION OF CONTAGION TO THE THEORY OF SPONTANEOUS GENERATION.--NEEDHAM AND SPALLANZANI.--THE DISCOVERY OF THE COMPOUND MICROSCOPE IN 1605.--THE PROOF THAT A LIVING ORGANISM IS THE CAUSE OF A DISEASE.--ANTHRAX.--THE DISCOVERY OF THE ANTHRAX BACILLUS IN 1851.--THE CULTIVATION OF THE BACILLUS BY KOCH.--THE MODE OF INFECTION.--THE WORK OF PASTEUR ON ANTHRAX.--THE IMPORTANCE OF THE DISEASE.

These are diseases which are caused by living things which enter the tissues of the body and, living at the expense of the body, produce injury. Such diseases play an important part in the life of man; the majority of deaths are caused directly or indirectly by infection. No other diseases have been so much studied, and in no other department of science has knowledge been capable of such direct application in promoting the health, the efficiency and the happiness of man. This knowledge has added years to the average length of life, it has rendered possible such great engineering works as the Panama Canal, and has contributed to the food supply by making habitation possible over large and productive regions of the earth, formerly uninhabitable owing to the prevalence of disease. It is not too much to say that our modern civilization is dependent upon this knowledge. The massing of the people in large cities, the factory life, the much greater social life, which are all prominent features of modern civilization, would be difficult or impossible without control of the infectious diseases. The rapidity of communication and the increased general movement of people, which have developed in equal ratio with the massing, would serve to extend widely every local outbreak of infection. The principles underlying fermentation and putrefaction which have been applied with great economic advantage to the preservation of food were many of them developed in the course of the study of the infectious diseases. Whether the development of the present civilization is for the ultimate advantage of man may perhaps be disputed, but medicine has made it possible.

The infectious diseases appearing in the form of great epidemics have been important factors in determining historical events, for they have led to the defeat of armies, the fall of cities and of nations. War is properly regarded as one of the greatest evils that can afflict a nation, since it destroys men in the bloom of youth, at the age of greatest service, and brings sorrow and care and poverty to many. But the most potent factor in the losses of war is not the deaths in battle but the deaths from disease. If we designate the lives lost in battle, the killed and the wounded who die, as 1, the loss of the German army from disease in 1870-71 was 1.5, that of the Russians in 1877-78 was 2.7, that of the French in Mexico was 2.8, that of the French in the Crimea 3.7, that of the English in Egypt 4.2. The total loss of the German army in 1870-71 from wounds and disease was 43,182 officers and men, and this seems a small number compared with the 129,128 deaths from smallpox in the same period in Prussia alone. In the Spanish American war there were 20,178 cases of typhoid fever with 1,580 deaths. In the South African war there were in the British troops 31,118 cases of typhoid with 5,877 deaths, and 5,149 deaths from other diseases while the loss in battle was 7,582. The Athenian plague which prevailed during the Peloponnesian war, 431-405 B.C., not only caused the death of Pericles, but according to Thucydides a loss of 4,800 Athenian soldiers, and brought about the downfall of the Athenian hegemony in Greece. In the Crimean war between 1853-56, 16,000 English, 80,000 French and 800,000 Russians died of typhus fever. The plague contributed as much as did the arms of the Turks to the downfall of Constantinople and the Eastern Empire in 1453. It was the plague which in 1348 overthrew Siena from her proud position as one of the first of the Italian cities and the rival of

Florence, and broke the city forever, leaving it as a phantom of its former glory and prosperity. The work on the great cathedral which had progressed for ten years was suspended, and when it was resumed it was upon a scale adjusted to the diminished wealth of the city, and the plan restricted to the present dimensions. As a little relief to the darkness the same plague saw the birth of the novel in the tales of Boccaccio, which were related to a delighted audience of the women who had fled from the plague in Florence to a rural retreat.

The knowledge which has come from the study of infectious disease has served also to broaden our conception of disease and has created preventive medicine; it has linked more closely to medicine such sciences as zoology and botany; it has given birth to the sciences of bacteriology and protozoology and in a way has brought all sciences more closely together. Above all it has made medicine scientific, and never has knowledge obtained been more quickening and stimulating to its pursuit.

Although the dimensions of this book forbid much reference to the historical development of a subject, some mention must still be made of the development of knowledge of the infectious diseases. It was early recognized that there were diseases which differed in character from those generally prevalent; large numbers of people were affected in the same way; the disease beginning with a few cases gradually increased in intensity until an acme was reached which prevailed for a time and the disease gradually disappeared. Such diseases were attributed to changes in the air, to the influence of planets or to the action of offended gods. The priests and charlatans who sought to excuse their inability to treat epidemics successfully were quick to affirm supernatural causes. Hippocrates (400 B.C.), with whom medicine may be said to begin, thought such diseases, even then called epidemics, were caused by the air; he says, "When many individuals are attacked by a disease at the same time, the cause must be sought in some agent which is common to all, something which everyone uses, and that is the air which must contain at this time something injurious." Aristotle recognized that disease was often conveyed by contact, and Varro (116-27 B.C.) advanced the idea that disease might be caused by minute organisms. He says, "Certain minute organisms develop which the eye cannot see, and which being disseminated in the air enter into the body by means of the mouth and nostrils and give rise to serious ailments." In spite of this hypothesis, which has proved to be correct, the belief became general that epidemics were due to putrefaction of the air brought about by decaying animal bodies, (this explaining the frequent association of epidemics and wars,) by emanations from swamps, by periods of unusual heat, etc.

With the continued study of epidemics the importance of contagion was recognized; it was found that epidemics differed in character and in the modes of extension. Some seemed to extend by contact with the sick, and in others this seemed to play no part; it was further found impossible in many cases to show evidence of air contamination, and contamination of the air by putrefactive material did not always produce disease. Most important was the recognition that single cases of diseases which often occurred in epidemic form might be present and no further extension follow; this led to the assumption in epidemics of the existence of some condition in addition to the cause, and which made the cause operative. In this way arose the theory of the epidemic constitution, a supposed peculiar condition of the body due to changes in the character of the air, or to the climate, or to changes in the interior of the earth as shown by earthquakes, or to the movements of planets; in consequence of this peculiar constitution there was a greater susceptibility to disease, but the direct cause might arise in the interior of the body or enter the body from without. The character of the disease which appeared in epidemic form, the "Genius epidemicus," was determined not by differences in the intrinsic cause, but by the type of constitution which prevailed at that time. The first epidemic of cholera which visited Europe in 1830-37 was for the most part referred to the existence of a peculiar epidemic constitution for which various causes were assigned. It was only when the second epidemic of this disease appeared in 1840 that the existence of some special virus or poison which entered the body was assumed.

Meanwhile, by the study of the material of disease knowledge was being slowly acquired which had much bearing on the causes. The first observations which tended to show that the causes were living were made by a learned Jesuit, Athanasius, in 1659. He found in milk, cheese, vinegar, decayed vegetables, and in the blood and secretions of cases of plague bodies, which he described as tiny worms and which he thought were due to putrefaction. He studied these objects with the simple lenses in use at that time, and there is little doubt that he did see certain of the larger organisms which are present in vinegar, cheese and decaying vegetables, and it is not impossible that he may have seen the animal and vegetable cells.

The first description of bacteria with illustrations showing their forms was given by Loewenhoeck, a linen dealer in Amsterdam in 1675. The fineness of the linen being determined by the number of threads in a given area, it is necessary to examine it with a magnifying lens, and he succeeded in perfecting a simple lens with which objects smaller than had been seen up to that time became visible. It must be added that he was probably endowed with very unusual acuteness of vision. He found in a drop of water, in the fluid in the intestines of frogs and birds, and in his evacuations, objects of great minuteness which differed from each other in form and size and in the peculiar motion which some of them possessed. In the year 1683 he presented to the Royal Society of London a paper describing a certain minute organism which he found in the tartar of his teeth. After these observations of Loewenhoeck became known to the world they quickly found application in disease, although the author had expressed himself very cautiously in this regard. The strongest exponent of the view of a living contagion was Plenciz, 1762, a physician of Vienna, basing his belief not only on the demonstration of minute organisms by Loewenhoeck which he was able to verify, but on certain shrewdly conceived theoretical considerations. He was the first to recognize the specificity of the epidemic diseases, and argued from this that each disease must have a specific cause. "Just as a certain plant comes from the seed of the same plant and not from any plant at will, so each contagious disease must be propagated from a similar disease and cannot be the result of any other disease." Further he says, "It is necessary to assume that during the prevalence of an epidemic the contagious material undergoes an enormous increase, and this is compatible only with the assumption that it is a living substance." But as is so often the case, speculation ran far ahead of the observations on which it is based. There was a long gap between the observations of Loewenhoeck and the theories of Plenciz, justified as these have been by present knowledge. In the spirit of speculation which was dominant in Europe and particularly in Germany in the latter half of the eighteenth and the first half of the nineteenth centuries, hypotheses did not stimulate research, but led to further speculations. As late as 1820 Ozanam expressed himself as follows: "Many authors have written concerning the animal nature of the contagion of disease; many have assumed it to be developed from animal substance, and that it is itself animal and possesses the property of life. I shall not waste time in refuting these absurd hypotheses." The theory of a living contagion was too simple, and not sufficiently related to the problems of the universe to serve the medical philosophers.

Knowledge of the minute organisms was slowly accumulating. The first questions to be determined were as to their nature and origin. How were they produced? Did they come from bodies of the same sort according to the general laws governing the production of living things, or did they arise spontaneously? a question which could not be solved by speculation but by experiment. The first experiments, by Needham, 1745, pointed to the spontaneous origin of the organisms. He enclosed various substances in carefully sealed watch crystals from which the air was excluded, and found that animalculi appeared in the substance, and argued from this that they developed spontaneously. In 1769, Spallanzani, a skilled experimental physiologist, in a brilliant series of experiments showed the imperfect character of Needham's work and the fallacy of his conclusions. Spallanzani placed fluids, which easily became putrid, in glass tubes, which he then hermetically sealed and boiled. He found that the fluid remained clear and unchanged; if, however, he broke the sealed point of such a tube and allowed the air to enter, putrefaction, or in some cases fermentation, of the contents took place. He concluded that boiling the substances destroyed the living germs which they contained, the sealed tubes prevented the air from entering, and when putrefaction or fermentation of the contents took place the organisms to which this was due, being contained in the air, entered from without. Objection was made to the conclusions of Spallanzani that heating the air in the closed tubes so changed its character as to prevent development of organisms in the contents. This objection was finally set aside by Pasteur, who showed that it was not necessary to seal the end of the tube before boiling, but it could be closed by a plug of cotton wool, which mechanically removed the organisms from the air which entered the tube, or if the tube were bent in the shape of a U and the end left open, organisms from the air could not pass into the tube against gravity when air movement within the tube was prevented by bending. The possibility of spontaneous generation cannot be denied, but that it takes place is against all human experience.

It was not possible to attain any considerable knowledge of the bacteria discovered by Loewenhoeck until more perfect instruments for studying them were devised. Lenses for studying objects were used in remote antiquity, but the compound microscope in which the image made by the lens is further magnified was not discovered until 1605, and when first made was so imperfect that the best simple lenses gave clearer definition. With the betterment of the microscope, increasing the magnifying power and the sharpness of the image of the object seen, it became possible to classify the minute organisms according to size and form and to study the separate species. The microscope has now reached such a degree of perfection that objects smaller than one one hundred thousandth of an inch in diameter can be clearly seen and photographed.

Great impetus was given to the biological investigation of disease by the discoveries which led to the formulation of the cell theory in 1840 and the brilliant work of Pasteur on fermentation,[1] but it was not until 1878 that it was definitely proved that a disease of cattle called anthrax was due to a species of bacteria. What should be regarded as such proof had been formulated by Henle in 1840. To prove that a certain sort of organism when found associated with a disease is the cause of the disease, three things are necessary:

1. The organism must always be found in the diseased animal and associated with the changes produced by the disease.

2. The organism so found must be grown outside of the body in what is termed pure cultures, that is, not associated with any other organisms, and for so long a time with constant transfers or new seedings that there can be no admixture of other products of the disease in the material in which it is grown.

3. The disease must be produced by inoculating a susceptible animal with a small portion of such a culture, and the organism shown in relation to the lesions so produced.

It is worth while to devote some attention to the disease anthrax. This occupies a unique position, in that it was the first of the infectious diseases to be scientifically investigated. In this investigation one fact after another was discovered and confirmed; some of these facts seemed to give clearer conceptions of the disease, others served to make it more obscure; new questions arose with each extension of knowledge; in the course of the work new methods of investigation were discovered; the sides of the arch were slowly and painfully erected by the work of many men, and finally one man placed the keystone and anthrax was for a long time the best known of diseases. Men whose reputation is now worldwide first became known by their work in this disease. It was a favorable disease for investigation, being a disease primarily of cattle, but occasionally appearing in man, and the susceptibility of laboratory animals made possible experimental study.

Anthrax is a disease of domestic cattle affecting particularly bovine cattle, horses and sheep, swine more rarely. The disease exists in practically all countries and has caused great economic losses. There are no characteristic symptoms of the disease; the affected cattle have high fever, refuse to eat, their pulse and respiration are rapid, they become progressively weaker, unable to walk and finally fall. The disease lasts a variable time; in the most acute cases animals may die in less than twenty-four hours, or the disease may last ten or fourteen days; recovery from the disease is rare and treatment has no effect. It does not appear in the form of epidemics, but single cases appear frequently or rarely, and there is seemingly no extension from case to case, animals in adjoining stalls to the sick are not more prone to infection than others of the herd. On examination after death the blood is dark and fluid, the spleen is greatly enlarged (one of the names of the disease "splenic fever" indicates the relation to the spleen) and there is often bloody fluid in the tissues.

Where the disease is prevalent there are numbers of human cases. Only those become infected who come into close relations with cattle, the infection most commonly taking place from small wounds or scratches made in skinning dead cattle or in handling hides. The wool of sheep who die of the disease finds its way into commerce, and those employed in handling the wool have a form of anthrax known as wool-sorters' disease in which lesions are found in the lungs, the organisms being mingled with the wool dust and inspired. In Boston occasional cases of anthrax appear in teamsters who are employed in handling and carrying hides. The disease in man is not so fatal as in cattle, for it remains local for a time at the site of infection, and this local disease can be successfully treated.

The beginning of our knowledge of the cause dates from 1851, when small rod-shaped bodies (Fig. 17) were found in the blood of the affected cattle, and by the work of a number of observers it was established that these bodies were constantly present. Nothing was known of their nature; some held that they were living organisms, others that they were formed in the body as a result of the disease. Next the causal relation of these bodies with the disease was shown and in several ways. The disease could be caused in other cattle by injecting blood containing the rods beneath the skin, certainly no proof, for the blood might have contained in addition to the rods something which was the real cause of the disease. Next it was shown that the blood of the unborn calf of a cow who died of the disease did not contain the rods, and the disease could not be produced by inoculating with the calf's blood although the blood of the mother was infectious. This was a very strong indication that the rods were the cause; the maternal and foetal blood are separated by a membrane through which fluids and substances in solution pass; but insoluble substances, even when very minutely subdivided, do not pass the membrane. If the cause were a poison in solution, the foetal blood would have been as toxic as the maternal. The blood of infected cattle was filtered through filters made of unbaked porcelain and having very fine pores which allowed only the blood fluid to pass, holding back both the blood corpuscles and the rods, and such filtered blood was found to be innocuous. It was further shown that the rods increased enormously in number in the infected animal, for the blood contained them in great numbers when but a fraction of a drop was used for inoculation. Attempts were also made with a greater or less degree of success to grow the rod shaped organisms or bacilli in various fluids, and the characteristic disease was produced by inoculating animals with these cultures; but it remained for Koch, 1878, who was at that time an obscure young country physician, to show the life history of the organism and to clear up the obscurity of the disease. Up to that time, although it had been shown that the rods or bacilli contained in the blood were living organisms and the cause of the disease, this did not explain the mode of infection; how the organisms contained in the blood passed to another animal, why the disease occurred on certain farms and the adjoining farms, particularly if they lay higher, were free. Koch showed that in the cultures the organisms grew out into long interlacing threads, and that in these threads spores which were very difficult to destroy developed at intervals; that the organisms grew easily in bouillon, in milk, in blood, and even in an infusion of hay made by soaking this in water. This explained, what had been an enigma before, how the fields became sources of infection. The infection did not spread from animal to animal by contact, but infection took place from eating grass or hay which contained either the bacilli or their spores. When a dead animal was skinned on the field, the bacilli contained in the blood escaped and became mingled with the various fluids which flowed from the body and in which they grew and developed spores. It was shown by Pasteur that even when a carcass was buried the earthworms brought spores developed in the body to the surface and deposited them in their casts, and in this way also the fields became infected. From such a spot of infected earth the spores could be washed by the rains over greater areas and would find opportunity to develop further and form new spores in puddles of water left on the fields, which became a culture medium by the soaking of the dead grass. The contamination of the fields was also brought about by spreading over them the accumulations of stable manure which contained the discharges of the sick cattle. The tendency of the disease to extend to lower-lying adjacent fields was due to the spores being washed from the upper fields to the lower by the spring freshets. Meanwhile Pasteur had discovered that by growing the organisms at higher temperatures than the animal body, it was possible to attenuate the virulence of the bacilli so that inoculations with these produced a mild form of the disease which rendered the inoculated animals immune to the fatal disease. The description of Pasteur's work on the disease as given in the account of his life by his son-in-law is fascinating.

Hides and wool taken from dead animals invariably contained the spores which could pass unharmed through some of the curing processes, and were responsible for some of the cases in man. Owing to the introduction of regulations which were based on the knowledge of the cause of the disease and the life history of the organism, together with the prophylactic inoculation devised by Pasteur, the incidence of the disease has been very greatly lessened. Looking at the matter from the lowest point of view, the money which has been saved by the control of the disease, as shown in its decline, has been many times the cost of all the work of the investigations which made the control possible. It is a greater satisfaction to know that many human lives have been saved, and that small farmers and shepherds have been the chief sharers in the economic benefits. The indirect benefits, however, which have resulted from the application of the knowledge of this disease, and the methods of investigation developed here, to the study of the infections more peculiar to man, are very much greater.

FOOTNOTE: [1] The interesting analogy between fermentation and infectious disease did not escape attention. A clear fluid containing in solution sugar and other constituents necessary for the life of the yeast cells will remain clear provided all living things within it have been destroyed and those in the air prevented from entering. If it be inoculated with a minute fragment of yeast culture containing a few yeast cells, for a time no change takes place; but gradually the fluid becomes cloudy, bubbles of gas appear in it and its taste changes. Finally it again becomes clear, a sediment forms at the bottom, and on re-inoculating it with yeast culture no fermentation takes place. The analogy is obvious, the fluid in the first instance corresponds with an individual susceptible to the disease, the inoculated yeast to the contagion from a case of transmissible disease, the fermentation to the illness with fever, etc., which constitutes the disease, the returning clearness of the fluid to the recovery, and like the fermenting fluid the individual is not susceptible to a new attack of the disease. It will be observed that during the process both the yeast and the material which produced the disease have enormously increased. Fermentation of immense quantities of fluid could be produced by the sediment of yeast cells at the bottom of the vessel and a single case of smallpox would be capable of infecting multitudes.

CHAPTER VI

CLASSIFICATION OF THE ORGANISMS WHICH CAUSE DISEASE.--BACTERIA: SIZE, SHAPE, STRUCTURE, CAPACITY FOR GROWTH, MULTIPLICATION AND SPORE FORMATION.--THE ARTIFICIAL CULTIVATION OF BACTERIA.--THE IMPORTANCE OF BACTERIA IN NATURE.--VARIATIONS IN BACTERIA.-- SAPROPHYTIC AND PARASITIC FORMS.--PROTOZOA.--STRUCTURE MORE COMPLICATED THAN THAT OF BACTERIA.--DISTRIBUTION IN NATURE.-- GROWTH AND MULTIPLICATION.-- CONJUGATION AND SEXUAL REPRODUCTION.--SPORE FORMATION.--THE NECESSITY FOR A FLUID ENVIRONMENT.--THE FOOD OF PROTOZOA.--PARASITISM.--THE ULTRA-MICROSCOPIC OR FILTERABLE--ORGANISMS.--THE LIMITATION OF THE MICROSCOPE.--PORCELAIN FILTERS TO SEPARATE ORGANISMS FROM A FLUID.-- FOOT AND MOUTH DISEASE PRODUCED BY AN ULTRA-MICROSCOPIC ORGANISM.-- OTHER DISEASES SO PRODUCED.--DO NEW DISEASES APPEAR?

The living organisms which cause the infectious diseases are classified under bacteria, protozoa, yeasts, moulds, and ultra-microscopic organisms. It is necessary to place in a separate class the organisms whose existence is known, but which are not visible under the highest powers of the microscope, and have not been classified. The yeasts and moulds play a minor part in the production of disease and cannot be considered in the necessary limitation of space.

[Illustration: FIG. 17.--VARIOUS FORMS OF BACTERIA, a, b, c, d, Round bacteria or cocci: (_a_) Staphylococci, organisms which occur in groups and a common cause of boils; (_b_) streptococci, organisms which occur in chains and produce erysipelas and more severe forms of inflammation; (_c_) diplococci, or paired organisms with a capsule, which cause acute pneumonia; (_d_) gonococci, with the opposed surfaces flattened, which cause gonorrhoea. e, f, g, h, Rod-shaped bacteria or bacilli: (_e_) diphtheria bacilli; (_f_) tubercle bacilli; (_g_) anthrax bacilli; (_h_) the same bacilli in cultures and producing spores; a small group of spores is shown. (_i_) Cholera spirill? (_j_) Typhoid bacilli. (_k_) Tetanus bacillus; i, j, k are actively motile, motion being effected by the small attached threads. (_l_) The screw-shaped spirochite which is the cause of syphilis.]

The bacteria (Fig. 17) are unicellular organisms and vary greatly in size, shape and capacity of growth. The smallest of the pathogenic or disease-producing bacteria is the influenza bacillus, 1/51000 of an inch in length and 1/102000 of an inch in thickness; and among the largest is a bacillus causing an animal disease which is 1/2000 of an inch in length and 1/25000 of an inch in diameter. Among the free-living non-pathogenic forms much larger examples are found. In shape bacteria are round, or rod-shaped, or spiral; the round forms are called micrococci, the rod-shaped bacilli and the spiral forms are called spirilli. A clearer idea of the size is possibly given by the calculation that a drop of water would contain one billion micrococci of the usual size. Their structure in a general way conforms with that of other cells. On the outside is a cell membrane which encloses cytoplasm and nucleus; the latter, however, is not in a single mass, but the nuclear material is distributed through the cell. Many of the bacteria have the power of motion, this being effected by small hair-like appendages or flagell?which may be numerous, projecting from all parts of the organisms or from one or both ends, the movement being produced by rapid lashing of these hairs. A bacterium grows until it attains the size of the species, when it divides by simple cleavage at right angles to the long axis forming two individuals. In some of the spherical forms division takes place alternately in two planes, and not infrequently the single individuals adhere, forming figures of long threads or chains or double forms. The rate of growth varies with the species and with the environment, and under the best conditions may be very rapid. A generation, that is, the interval between divisions, has been seen to take place in twenty minutes. At this rate of growth from a single cholera bacillus sixteen quadrillion might arise in a single day. Such a rate of growth is extremely improbable under either natural or artificial conditions, both from lack of food and from the accumulation in the fluid of waste products which check growth. Many species of bacteria in addition to this simple mode of multiplication form spores which are in a way analogous to the seeds of higher plants and are much more resistant than the simple or vegetative forms; they endure boiling water and even higher degrees of dry heat for a considerable time before they are destroyed. When these spores are placed in conditions favorable for bacterial life, the bacterial cells grow out from them and the usual mode of multiplication continues. This capacity for spore formation is of great importance, and until it was discovered by Cohn in 1876, many of the conditions of disease and putrefaction could not be explained. Spores, as the seeds of plants, often seem to be produced when the conditions are unfavorable; the bacterium then changes into this form, which under natural conditions is almost indestructible and awaits better days.

The bacteria are divided into species, the classification being based on their forms, on the mode of growth, the various substances which they produce and their capacity for producing disease. The differentiation of species in bacteria is based chiefly upon their properties, there being too little difference in form and size to distinguish species. The introduction of methods of culture was followed by an immediate advance of our knowledge concerning them. This method consists in the use of fluid and solid substances which contain the necessary salts and other ingredients for their food, and in or on which they are planted. The use of a solid or gelatinous medium for growth has greatly facilitated the separation of single species from a mixture of bacteria; a culture fluid containing sufficient gelatine to render it solid when cooled is sown with the bacteria to be tested by placing in it while warm and fluid, a small portion of material containing the bacteria, and after being thoroughly mixed the fluid is poured on a glass plate and allowed to cool. The bacteria are in this way separated, and each by its growth forms a single colony which can be further tested. It is self-evident that all culture material must be sterilized by heat before using, and in the manipulations care must be exercised to avoid contamination from the air. The refraction index of the bacterial cell is so slight that the microscopic study is facilitated or made possible by staining them with various aniline dyes. Owing to differences in the cell material the different species of bacteria show differences in the facility with which they take the color and the tenacity with which they retain it, and this also forms a means of species differentiation. The interrelation of science is well shown in this, for it was the discovery of the aniline dyes in the latter half of the nineteenth century which made the fruitful study of bacteria possible.

From the simplicity of structure it is not improbable that the bacteria are among the oldest forms of life, and all life has become adapted to their presence. They are of universal distribution; they play such an important part in the inter-relations of living things that it is probable life could not continue without them, at least not in the present way. They form important food for other unicellular organisms which are important links in the chain; they are the agents of decomposition, by which the complex substances of living things are reduced to elementary substances and made available for use; without them plant life would be impossible, for it is by their instrumentality that material in the soil is so changed as to be available as plant food; by their action many of the important foods of man, often those especially delectable, are produced; they are constantly with us on all the surfaces of the body; masses live on the intestinal surfaces and the excrement is largely composed of bacteria. It has been said that life would be impossible without bacteria, for the accumulation of the carcasses of all animals which have died would so encumber the earth as to prevent its use; but the folly of such speculation is shown by the fact that animals would not have been there without bacteria. It has been shown, however, that the presence of bacteria in the intestine of the higher animals is not essential for life. The coldest parts of the ocean are free from those forms which live in the intestines, and fish and birds inhabiting these regions have been found free from bacteria; it has also been found possible to remove small animals from their mother by Caesarian section and to rear them for a few weeks on sterilized food, showing that digestion and nutrition may go on without bacteria.

Certain species of bacteria are aerobic, that is, they need free oxygen for their growth; others are anaerobic and will not grow in the presence of oxygen. Most of the bacteria which produce disease are facultative, that is, they grow either with or without oxygen; but certain of them, as the bacillus of tetanus, are anaerobic. There is, of course, abundance of oxygen in the blood and tissues, but it is so combined as to be unavailable for the bacteria. Bacteria may further be divided into those which are saprophytic or which find favorable conditions for life outside of the body, and the parasitic. Many are exclusively parasitic or saprophytic, and many are facultative, both conditions of living being possible. It has been found possible by varying in many ways the character of the culture medium and temperature to grow under artificial conditions outside of the body most, if not all, of the bacteria which cause disease. Thus, such bacteria as tubercle bacilli and the influenza bacillus can be cultivated, but they certainly would not find natural conditions which would make saprophytic growth possible.

Bacteria may be very sensitive to the presence of certain substances in the fluid in which they are growing. Growth may be inhibited by the smallest trace of some of the metallic salts, as corrosive sublimate, although the bacteria themselves are not destroyed. If small pieces of gold foil be placed on the surface of prepared jelly on which bacteria have been planted, no growth will take place in the vicinity of the gold foil.

Variations can easily be produced in bacteria, but they do not tend to become established. In certain of the bacterial species there are strains which represent slight variations from the type but which are not sufficient to constitute new species. If the environment in which bacteria are living be unusual and to a greater or less degree unfavorable, those individuals in the mass with the least power of adaptibility will perish, those more resistant and with greater adaptability will survive and propagate; and the peculiarity being transmitted a new strain will arise characterized by this adaptability. Bacteria with slight adaptability to the environment of the tissues and fluids of the animal body can, by repeated inoculations, become so adapted to the new environment as to be in a high degree pathogenic. In such a process the organisms with the least power of adaptation are destroyed and new generations are formed from those of greater power of adaptation. When bacteria are caused to grow in a new environment they may acquire new characteristics. The anthrax bacilli find the optimum conditions for growth at the temperature of the animal body, but they will grow at temperatures both above and below this. Pasteur found that by gradually increasing the temperature they could be grown at one hundred and ten degrees. When grown at this temperature they were no longer so virulent and produced in animals a mild non-fatal form of anthrax which protected the animal when inoculated with the virulent strain. The well known variations in the character of disease, shown in differences in severity and ease of transmission, seen in different years and in different epidemics, may be due to many conditions, but probably variation in the infecting organisms is the most important.

The protozoa, like the bacteria, are unicellular organisms and contain a nucleus as do all cells. They vary in size from forms seen with difficulty under the highest power of the microscope to forms readily seen with the unaided eye. Their structure in general is more complex than is the structure of bacteria, and many show extreme differentiation of parts of the single cells, as a firm exterior surface or cuticle, an internal skeleton, organs of locomotion, mouth and digestive organs and organs of excretion. They are more widely distributed than are the bacteria, and found from pole to pole in all oceans and in all fresh water. There are many modes of multiplication, and these are often extremely complicated. The most general mode and one which is common to all is by simple division; a modification of this is by budding in which projections or buds form on the body and after separation become new organisms. In other cases spores form within the cell which become free and develop further into complete organisms. These simple modes of multiplication often alternate in the same organism with sexual differentiation and conjugation. There is never a permanent sexual differentiation, but the sexual forms develop from a simple and non-sexual organism. Usually the sexual forms develop only in a special environment; thus the protozoon which in man is the cause of malaria, multiplies in the human blood by simple division, but in the body of the mosquito multiplication by sexual differentiation takes place. Under no conditions is multiplication so rapid as with the bacteria, and in general the simpler the form of organism the more rapid is the multiplication. It is common to all of the protozoa to develop forms which have great powers of resistance, this being due in some cases to encystment, in which condition a resistant membrane is formed on the outside, in others to the production of spores. A fluid environment is essential to the life of the protozoa, but the resistant forms can endure long periods of dryness or other unfavorable environmental conditions. The universal distribution of the protozoa is due to this; the spores or cysts can be carried long distances by the wind and develop into active forms when they reach an environment which is favorable. Their distribution in water depends upon the amount of organic material this contains. In pure drinking water there may be very few, but in stagnant water they are very numerous, living not on the organic material in solution in this, but on the bacteria which find in such fluid favorable conditions for existence. The food of protozoa consists chiefly of other organisms, particularly bacteria, and they are classed with the animals. The protozoa are the most widely distributed and the most universal of the parasites. The infectious diseases which they produce in man, although among the most serious are less in number than those produced by bacteria. So marked is the tendency to parasitism that they are often parasitic for each other, smaller forms entering into and living upon the larger. Variation does not seem to be so marked in the protozoa as in the bacteria, though this is possibly due to our greater ignorance of them as a class. We are not able, except in rare instances, to grow them in pure culture, and study innumerable generations under changes in the environment, as the bacteria have been studied.

If we regard the living things on earth from the narrow point of view as to whether they are necessary or useless or hostile to man, the protozoa must be regarded as about the least useful members of the biological society. It is very possible that such a conclusion is due to ignorance; so closely are all living things united, so dependent is one form of cell activity upon other forms that it is impossible to foretell the result of the removal of a link. The protozoa do not seem to be as necessary for the life of man as are the bacteria; they produce many of the diseases of man, many of the diseases of animals on which man depends for food; they cause great destruction in plant life, and in the soil they feed upon the useful bacteria. It is well to remember, however, that fifty years ago several of the organs of the body whose activity we now recognize as furnishing substances necessary for life were regarded as useless members and, since they became the seat of tumors, as dangerous members of the body. The only organ which now seems to come into such a class is the vermiform appendix, and its lowly position among organs is due merely to an unhappy accident of development.

The class of organisms known as the filterable viruses or the ultra-microscopic or the invisible organisms have a special interest in many ways.

The limitation in the power of the microscope for the study of minute objects is due not to a defect in the instrument but to the length of the wave of light. It is impossible to see clearly under the microscope using white light, objects which are smaller in diameter than the length of the wave which gives a limit of 0.5? or 1/125,000 of an inch. By using waves of shorter length, as the ultra-violet light, objects of 0.1? or 1/250000 of an inch can be seen; but as these methods depend upon photography for the demonstration of the object the study is difficult. The presence of objects still smaller than 0.1 m. can be detected in a fluid by the use of the dark field illumination and the ultra-microscope, the principle of which is the direction of a powerful oblique ray of light into the field of the microscope. The objects are not visible as such, but the dispersion of the light by their presence is seen.

The demonstration that infectious diseases were produced by organisms so small as to be beyond demonstration with the best microscopes was made possible by showing, that some fluid from a diseased animal was infectious; and capable of producing the disease when inoculated into a susceptible animal. The fluid was then filtered through porcelain filters which were known to hold back all objects of the size of the smallest bacteria and the disease produced by inoculating with the clear filtrate. There are a number of such filters of different degrees of porosity manufactured, and they are often used to procure pure water for drinking, for which use they are more or less, generally however, less efficacious. The filter has the form of a hollow cylinder and the liquid to be filtered is forced through it under pressure. For domestic use the filter is attached by its open end to the water tap and the pressure from the mains forces the water through it. In laboratory uses, denser filters of smaller diameters are used, and the filter is surrounded by the fluid to be tested. The open end of the filter passes into a vessel from which the air is exhausted and filtration takes place from without inward. The test of the effectiveness of the filter is made by adding to the filtering fluid some very minute and easily recognizable bacteria and testing the filtrate for their presence. These filters have been studied microscopically by grinding very thin sections and measuring the diameter of the spaces in the material. These are very numerous, and from 1/25000 to 1/1000 of an inch in diameter, spaces which would allow bacteria to pass through, but they are held back by the very fine openings between the spaces and by the tortuosity of the intercommunications. When the coarser of such filters have been long in domestic service in filtering drinking water, bacteria may grow in and through them giving greater bacterial content to the supposed bacteria-free filtrate than in the filtering water.

That an animal disease was due to such a minute and filterable organism was first shown by Loeffler in 1898 for the foot and mouth disease of cattle. This is one of the most infectious and easily communicable diseases. The lesions of the disease take the form of blisters which form on the lips and feet and in the mouths of cattle, and inoculation with minute quantities of the fluid in the blisters produces the disease. Loeffler filtered the fluid through porcelain filters, hoping to obtain a material which inoculated into other cattle would render them immune, and to his surprise found that the typical disease was produced by inoculating with the filtrate. Naturally the first idea was that the disease was caused by some soluble poison and not by a living organism, but this was disproved in a number of ways. The most powerful poison known is obtained from cultures of the tetanus bacillus of which 0.000,000,1 of a gram (one gram is 15.43 grains) kills a mouse, or one gram kills ten million mice. Loeffler found that 1/30 gram of the contents of the vesicles killed a calf of two hundred kilograms weight, and assuming that the essential poison was present in the fluid in one part to five hundred it would be several hundred times more powerful than the tetanus poison. Further, the disease produced by inoculation of the filtrate was itself inoculable and could be transmitted from animal to animal. It was also found that when the virus was filtered several times it ceased to be inoculable, showing that each time the fluid was passed through the filter some of the minute organisms contained in it were held back.

It is not known whether these organisms belong to the bacteria or protozoa, and naturally nothing is known as to their form, size and structure. Up to the present about twenty diseases are known to be due to a filterable virus, and among these are some of the most important for animals and for man. Among the human diseases, yellow fever, poliomyelitis, and dengue are so produced; of the animal diseases in addition to foot and mouth disease, pleuropneumonia, cattle plague, African horse sickness, several diseases of fowls and the mosaic disease of the tobacco plant have all been shown to be due to a filterable virus. Of these organisms the largest is that which produces pleuropneumonia in cattle, and this alone has been cultivated. It gives a slight opacity to the culture fluids, and when magnified two thousand diameters appears as a minute spiral or round or stellate organism having a variety of forms. Its size is such that it passes the coarse, but is held back by the finer, filters and it is possible that this does not belong to the same class with the others.[1] The diseases produced by the filterable viruses taken as a class show much similarity. They run an acute course, are severe, and the immunity produced by the attack endures for a long time.

Considered in its biological relations, infection is the adaptation of an organism to the environment which the body of the host offers. It is rather singular that variations in organisms represented by such adaptation do not more frequently arise, in which case new diseases would frequently occur. It cannot be denied that new diseases appear, but there is no certain evidence that they do, and there is equally no evidence that diseases disappear. From the meagre descriptions of diseases, usually of the epidemic type, which have come down to us from the past, it is difficult to recognize many of the diseases described. The single diseases are recognized by comparing the causes, the lesions and the symptoms with those of other diseases, and new diseases are constantly being separated off from other diseases having more or less common features. Many new diseases have been recognized and named, but it is always more than probable that previously they were confounded with other diseases. Smallpox is such a characteristic disease that one would think it would have been recognized as an entity from the beginning, but although the description of some of the epidemics in remote times conform more or less to the disease as we know it, the first accurate description is in the eighth century by the Arabian physician Rhazes. Cerebro-spinal meningitis was not recognized as a separate disease until 1803, diphtheria not until 1826, and the separation between typhoid and typhus fever was not made before 1840. Nor is it sure that any diseases have disappeared, although there seems to have been a change in the character of many. It is difficult to reconcile leprosy as it appears now with the universal horror felt towards it, due to the persistence of the old traditions. It is possible, however, that the disease has not changed its character, but that such diseases as smallpox, syphilis, and certain forms of tuberculosis were formerly confounded with leprosy, thus giving a false idea of its prevalence.

In certain cases the adaptation of the organism is for a narrow environment; for example, the parasitism may extend to a simple species only, in others the adaptation may extend to a number of genera. In certain cases the adaptation is mutual, extending to both parasite and host and resulting in symbiosis, and this condition may be advantageous for both. Certain of the protozoa harbor within them cells of alg?utilizing to their own advantage the green chlorophil of the alg?in obtaining energy from sunlight and in turn giving sustenance to the alg? Although the alg?are useful guests, when they become too numerous the protozoan devours them. It is evident that symbiosis is the most favorable condition for the existence of the parasite, and an injurious action exerted by the parasite on the host unfavorable. The death of the host is an unfortunate incident from the parasite's point of view in that it is deprived of habitation and food supply, being placed in the same unfortunate situation as may befall a social parasite by the death of his host.

FOOTNOTE: [1] Flexner has recently succeeded in isolating and cultivating the organism of poliomyelitis, but the organism is so small that its classification is not possible.

CHAPTER VII

THE NATURE OF INFECTION.--THE INVASION OF THE BODY FROM ITS SURFACES.--THE PROTECTION OF THESE SURFACES.--CAN BACTERIA PASS THROUGH AN UNINJURED SURFACE.--INFECTION FROM WOUNDS.--THE WOUNDS IN MODERN WARFARE LESS PRONE TO INFECTION.--THE RELATION OF TETANUS TO WOUNDS CAUSED BY THE TOY PISTOL.--THE PRIMARY FOCUS OR ATRIUM OF INFECTION.--THE DISSEMINATION OF BACTERIA IN THE BODY.--THE DIFFERENT DEGREES OF RESISTANCE TO BACTERIA SHOWN BY THE VARIOUS ORGANS.--MODE OF ACTION OF BACTERIA.--TOXIN PRODUCTION.--THE RESISTANCE OF THE BODY TO BACTERIA.--CONFLICT BETWEEN PARASITE AND HOST.--ON BOTH SIDES MEANS OF OFFENSE AND DEFENSE.--PHAGOCYTOSIS.--THE DESTRUCTION OF BACTERIA BY THE BLOOD.--THE TOXIC BACTERIAL DISEASES.--TOXIN AND ANTITOXIN.--IMMUNITY.--THE THEORY OF EHRLICH.

As has been said, infection consists in the injury of the body by living organisms which enter it. The body is in relation to the external world by its surfaces only, and organisms must enter it by some one of these surfaces. It is true that the bacteria in the intestine--either those normally present or unusual varieties--may, under certain circumstances, produce substances which are injurious when absorbed; but this is not infection, and is analogous to any other sort of poisoning. Each surface of the body has its own bacterial flora. Organisms live on the surface either on matter which is secreted by the surface or they use up an inappreciable amount of body material. Many of these bacteria are harmless, some are protective, producing by their growth such changes in the surface fluids that these become hostile to the existence of other and pathogenic forms. The surfaces also frequently harbor pathogenic organisms which await some condition to arise which will permit them to effect entrance into the tissues.

The surfaces of the body protect from invasion to a greater or less degree. The skin protects by the impervious horny layer on the outside, the external cells of which are dead and constantly being thrown off. Bacteria are always found on and in this layer, but the conditions for growth here are not very favorable and the surface is constantly cleansed by desquamation. The new cells to supply the loss are produced in the deepest layer of the epidermis, and the movement of cells and fluids takes place from within outwards. The protection is less perfect about the hairs and the sweat glands. Infection by the route of the sweat glands is, however, uncommon, for the sweat is a fluid unfavorable for bacterial growth and the flow acts mechanically in washing away organisms which may have entered the ducts. Infection by the route of the hair follicles is common. There is no mechanical cleansing as by the sweat, the space around the hair is large and the accumulated secretion of the hair glands and the desquamated cells furnish a material in which bacteria may grow. Growing as a mass in this situation, they may produce sufficient toxic material to destroy adjacent living cells and thus effect entrance. Infection from the eye is not common, the surface, though moist, is smooth; the eyelashes around the margin of the lids give some mechanical protection from the entrance of bacteria contained in dust, and the movements of the lids and the constant and easily accelerated secretion of tears act mechanically in removing foreign substances. It is possible that the mechanical cleansing of the skin by the daily bath may have some action in preventing infection.

The internal surfaces are much more exposed to attack and the protection is not so efficient. The moisture of these surfaces is both a protection and a source of danger. It protects by favoring the lodgment near the orifices of organisms which are in the inspired air, for when bacteria touch a moist surface they cannot be raised from this and carried further by air currents. The moisture is a source of danger in that it favors the growth of bacteria which lodge on the surface. The respiratory surface which is most exposed to infection from the air is further protected by the cilia, which are fine hair-like processes covering the cells of the surface and which by their constant motion sweep out fine particles of all sorts which lodge upon them. The cavity of the mouth harbors large numbers of organisms, many of them pathogenic. It forms a depot from which bacteria may pass to communicating surfaces and infection from these may result. Food particles collect in the mouth and provide culture material, and there are many crypts and irregularities of surface which oppose mechanical cleaning. Infection of the middle ear, the most common cause of deafness, takes place by means of the Eustachian tube which connects the cavity of the ear with the mouth. Organisms from the mouth can extend into the various large salivary glands by means of the ducts and give rise to infections. The tonsils, particularly in children, provide a favorable surface for infection. The mucous surface extends into these forming deep pockets lined with very thin epithelium, and in these d 閣 ris of all sorts accumulates and provides material favorable for bacterial growth.

The lungs at first sight seem to offer the most favorable surface for infection. The surface, ninety-seven square yards, is enormous; it is moist, the epithelial covering is so thin as to give practically no mechanical protection, large amounts of air constantly pass in and out, and the surface is in contact with this. They are protected from infection in many ways. The tubes or bronchi by which the air passes into and from the lungs are covered with cilia; the surface area of these tubes constantly enlarges as they branch, the sum of the diameters of the small tubes being many times greater than that of the windpipe, and this enlargement by retarding the motion of the air favors the lodgment of particles on the surface whence they are removed by the action of the cilia. The entering air is also brought closely in contact with a moist surface at the narrow opening of the larynx. That bacteria and other foreign substances can enter the lungs in spite of these guards is shown not only by the infections which take place here, but also by the large amount of black carbon deposited in them from the soot contained in the air.

Infection rarely takes place from the surface of the gullet or oesophagus which leads from the mouth to the stomach. This is due to the smoothness of the surface and to the rapidity with which food passes over it. Infection by the stomach also is rare, for this contains a strong acid secretion which destroys many of the bacteria which are taken in with the food. It is found impossible to infect animals with cholera unless the acidity of the stomach contents be neutralized by an alkali. Many organisms, although their growth in the stomach is inhibited, are not destroyed there and pass into the intestines, where the conditions for infection are more favorable. This large and very irregular surface is bathed in fluid which is a good culture medium and but a single layer of cells covers it. The organisms which cause many of the infectious diseases in both man and animals find entrance by means of the alimentary canal, as cholera, dysentery, typhoid fever, chicken cholera, hog cholera.

Infection by the genito-urinary surface is comparatively rare. The surface openings are usually closed, and the discharge of urine has a mechanical cleansing effect. The wide tube of the vagina is further protected by a normal bacterial flora which produces conditions hostile to other and pathogenic bacteria. The most common infections are the sexual diseases, which are due to organisms which find favorable conditions for growth in and on the surface and which are conveyed from a similar surface by sexual contact.

It remains a question whether bacteria can penetrate an intact surface producing no injury at the point of entrance and be carried by the lymph or blood into internal organs where they produce disease. Internal infections are often found with seemingly intact body surfaces, but it is impossible to exclude the presence of minute or microscopic surface injuries by which the organisms may have entered. It is also possible that a slight injury at the point of entrance may heal so completely as to leave no trace.

The chief danger from wounds is that their surfaces may become infected. Death from wounds is due more frequently to infection than to the actual injury represented by the wounds. Much depends upon the character of the wound. Infection of clean wounds which are made by a sharp cutting instrument and from which there is abundant h鎚orrhage with sealing of the edges of the wound by clotted blood, rarely happens. Typical wounds of this sort are often made in shaving, and infection of such wounds is extraordinarily rare. If, with the wound, pathogenic organisms are placed in the tissue, or foreign substances such as bits of clothing are carried in with a bullet, for example, or if the instrument causing the wound be of such a character as to produce extensive lacerations of tissue, infection is more apt to occur. The less frequency of infection in modern wars is in part due to the simpler character of the wounds and in part to the fact that modern fixed ammunition is practically free from germs. The old spear-head, the arrow, the cross bow bolt, had little regard for the probabilities of infection. Whether infection follows a wound depends both upon the entry of pathogenic organisms and upon these finding in the tissues suitable opportunities for growth. In wounds in which there is much laceration of tissue organisms find the most favorable conditions for development. The very slight wounds produced by the exploded cap in the toy pistol give suitable conditions for the development of the bacillus which produces tetanus or lockjaw. The deaths of children from lockjaw following a Fourth of July celebration have often exceeded the total deaths in a Central American revolution. The tetanus bacillus is a widely distributed organism, whose normal habitat is in the soil and which is usually present on the dirty hands of little boys. The toy-pistol wounds are made by small bits of paper or metal being driven into the skin by the explosion of the cap. The wound is of little moment, the surface becomes closed, and a bit of foreign substance, a few dead cells and the tetanus bacilli from the surface remain enclosed and in a few days the fatal disease develops. Infection of the surfaces of old wounds such as the surface of an ulcer takes place with difficulty. Large numbers of leucocytes which give protection by phagocytosis are constantly passing to the surface, and there is also a constant stream of fluid towards the surface. On such a surface there may be an abundant growth of pathogenic organisms, but no infection results.

In most infections there is a focus where the infectious organisms are localized; this may correspond to the point of entrance on a surface or it may be in the interior of the body, the organisms being deposited there after entrance. At this primary localization, the atrium of infection,[1] the organisms multiply and from this point further invasion takes place. Many secondary foci may be formed in the organs by distribution of the organisms, or there may be infection of the blood and fluids of the body. The injuries which are produced depend upon the nature of the infecting organisms. The most common lesion consists in the death of the tissue about the infecting organisms. In most cases the sum of the changes are so characteristic that from them the nature of the infection is easily determined, and these changes often give names to the disease; thus tuberculosis is a disease characterized by the formation of tubercles or little nodules in the body. The situation of the foci of disease is determined by many conditions, the most important being the varying resistance of the different organs of the body to the growth of bacteria. Certain organs, such as the central nervous system, the muscles, the testicles and the ovaries, have a high resistance to the growth of bacteria. The disease may be localized in certain organs because only in these do the bacteria find favorable conditions for growth. In spite of a high general resistance to infection the lesions in chronic glanders are most marked in the muscles, those of poliomyelitis in the spinal cord. There are few bacterial diseases which are localized in the blood, but many of the diseases caused by protozoa have this localization. In every infection some organisms enter the blood, which acts as a carrier and deposits them in the organs.

Bacteria cause disease by producing substances called toxines which are poisonous to the cells, and of which two sorts are distinguished. One form of toxines is produced by the bacteria as a sort of secretion, and is formed both in the body and when the bacteria are growing in cultures. Substances of this character, many of them highly poisonous, are produced both by animals and plants. They may serve the purpose both of offence and defence, as in the case of the snake venom, and in other cases they seem to benefit their producers in no way whatever, and may even be injurious to them. After the different cereals have been grown for succeeding years in the same place, growth finally diminishes not from the exhaustion of the soil, but from the accumulation in it of substances produced by the plants. Beneath certain trees, as the Norway maple, grass will not grow, and it has been shown that the tree produces substances which inhibit the growth of grass. When bacteria are grown in a culture flask, growth ceases long before the nutritive material has been consumed, from the accumulation of waste products in the fluid. The other class of toxic substances, called endotoxines, are not secretion products, but are contained in the bacterial substance and become active by the destruction and disintegration of the bacteria. They can be artificially produced by grinding up masses of bacteria, and in the body the destruction and solution of bacteria which is constantly taking place sets them free. The toxines and the endotoxines are of an albuminous nature, and act only when they come in contact with the living cells within the body. When taken into the alimentary canal they are either not absorbed or so changed by the digestive fluids as to be innocuous. Many of the ordinary food substances, even a material apparently so simple as the white of an egg, are highly injurious if they reach the tissues in an unchanged form.

By means of these substances the bacteria produce such changes in their environment within the body that this becomes adapted to their parasitic existence. In symbiosis the bacteria probably undergo changes by which they become adapted to the environment, and in parasitism the environment becomes adapted to them. In the same way man can change his immediate environment by means of clothing, artificial heating, etc., and adapt it to his needs; or by hardening his body he can adapt it to the environment. The pathogenic bacterium finds the living tissue hostile, its cells devour him, the tissue fluids destroy him, and by means of the toxines he changes the environment from that of living to dead tissue, or in other ways so alters it that it is no longer hostile. The parasite has also means of passive defence comparable to the armor of the warrior in the past. It may form a protective mantle called a capsule around itself, which serves to protect it from the action of the body fluids. Such capsule formation is a very common thing in the pathogenic organisms, and they are found only when these are growing in the body and do not appear in cultures (Fig. 17-c).

It is evident that just as the parasite has his weapons of offence and defence so has the host, otherwise there would be no recovery from infectious diseases. Although many of the infectious diseases have a high mortality, which in rare instances reaches one hundred per cent, the majority do recover. In certain cases the recovery is attended by immunity, the individual being protected to a greater or less degree from a recurrence of the same disease. The immunity is never absolute; it may last for a number of years only, and usually, if the disease be again acquired, the second attack is milder than the primary. Probably the most enduring immunity is in smallpox, although cases are known of two and even three attacks; the immunity is high in scarlet fever, measles, mumps and typhoid fever. The immunity from diphtheria is short, and in pneumonia, although there must be a temporary immunity, future susceptibility to the disease is probably increased. In certain cases the immunity is only local; the focus of disease heals because the tissue there has evolved means of protection from the parasite, but if any other part of the body be infected, the disease pursues the usual course. A boil, for example, is frequently followed by the appearance of similar boils in the vicinity due to the infection of the skin by the micrococci from the first boil, which by dressings, etc., have become spread over the surface.

The natural methods of defence of the host against the parasites have formed the main subject in the study of the infectious diseases for the last twenty years. Speculation in this territory has been rife and most of it fruitless, but by patient study of disease in man and by animal experimentation there has been gradually evolved a sum of knowledge which has been applied in many cases to the treatment of infectious diseases with immense benefit. Research was naturally turned to this subject, for it was evident that the processes by which the protection of the body was brought about must be known before there could be a really rational method of treatment directed towards the artificial induction of such processes, or hastening and strengthening those which were taking place. Previous to knowledge of the bacteria, their mode of life, their methods of infection and knowledge of the defences of the body, most of the methods of prevention and treatment of the infectious diseases was based largely on conjecture, the one brilliant exception being the discovery of vaccination by Jenner in 1798.

The host possesses the passive defences of the surfaces which have already been considered. The first theories advanced in explanation of immunity were influenced by what was known of fermentation. One, the exhaustion theory, assumed that in the course of disease substances contained in the body and necessary for the growth of the bacteria became exhausted and the bacteria died in consequence. Another, the theory of addition, assumed that in the course of the disease substances inimical to the bacteria were formed. Both these theories were inadequate and not in accord with what was known of the physiology of the body. The most general mode of defence is by phagocytosis, the property which many cells have of devouring and digesting solid substances (Fig. 16-p). Although this had been known to take place in the amoeb?and other unicellular organisms, the wide extent of the process and its importance in immunity was first recognized by Metschnikoff in 1884 and the phagocytic theory of immunity advanced and defended by a brilliant series of experiments by Metschnikoff and his pupils conducted in the Pasteur Institute. Metschnikoff's first observations were made on the daphnea, a small animalcule just visible to the naked eye which lives in fresh water. The structure of the organism is simple, consisting of an external and internal surface between which there is a space, the body cavity; daphne?are transparent and can be studied under the microscope while living. Metschnikoff observed that certain of them in the aquarium gradually lost their transparency and died, and examining these he found they were attacked by a species of fungus having long, thin spores. These spores were taken into the intestine with other food; they penetrated the thin wall of the intestine, passed into the body cavity, multiplied there, and in consequence the animal died. In many cases, however, those penetrating became enclosed in cells which the body cavity contains and which correspond with the leucocytes of the blood; in these the spores were digested and destroyed. The daphne?in which this took place recovered from the infection. Here was a case in which all the stages of an infectious disease could be directly followed under the microscope, and the whole process was simple in comparison with infections in the higher animals. The pathogenic organism was known, the manner and site of invasion was clear, it was also evident that if the multiplication of the parasite was unchecked the animal died, but if the parasite was opposed by the body cells and destroyed the animal recovered. The studies were carried further into the diseases of the higher animals, and it was found the leucocytes in these played the same part as did the cells in the body cavity of the daphnea. The introduction of bacteria into certain animals was followed by their destruction within cells and no disease resulted; if this did not take place, the bacteria multiplied and produced disease. Support also was given the theory by the demonstration at about the same time that in most of the infectious diseases the leucocytes of the blood became increased in number,--that in pneumonia, for instance, instead of the usual number of eight thousand in a cubic millimeter of blood, there were often thirty thousand or even fifty thousand. At about the same time also chemotaxis, or the action of chemical substances in attracting or repelling organisms, excited attention, and all these facts together became woven into the theory. It was soon seen, however, that this theory, based as it was on observation and supported by the facts observed, was not, at least in its first crude form, capable of general application. Many animals have natural immunity to certain diseases; they do not have the disease under natural conditions, nor do they acquire the disease when the organisms causing it are artificially introduced into their tissues by inoculation. Such natural immunity seemed to be unconnected with defence by phagocytosis, for the leucocytes of the animal might or might not have phagocytic reaction to the particular organisms to which the animal was immune. It was also seen that recovery from infection in certain diseases was unconnected with phagocytosis. It had also been demonstrated, by German observers chiefly, that the serum of the blood, the colorless fluid in which the corpuscles float, was itself destructive, and that in an animal rendered immune to a special bacterium the destructive action of the serum on that organism was greatly increased. In this hostile serum the bacteria often became clumped together in masses, the bodies became swollen, broken up, and finally disintegrated. This property of the serum was described as due to a substance in the serum called alexine, which in the immune animal became greatly increased in amount. It was even denied by some that phagocytosis of living bacteria took place, and that all those included in the cells were dead, having been destroyed in the first instance by the serum. The strife became a national one between the French and Germans,--on the one side in France the phagocytic theory was defended, and in Germany, on the other, the theory of serum immunity. The mass of experimental work which poured from the laboratories of the two countries in attack and defence became so great that it could not easily be followed. It had a good influence because, without the stimulation of this national rivalry, the knowledge which gradually arose from this work would not have been so quickly acquired. It is interesting that the mode of action of the serum in destroying bacteria was demonstrated not by a German but by Bordet, a French observer and a pupil of Metschnikoff. He showed that the serum contained two distinct substances, each necessary for the destructive action. The separate action of these substances can be studied since one is thermolabile, or destroyed by heating the serum to one hundred and thirty-three degrees; the other thermostabile, or capable of withstanding a greater degree of heat. These substances are known only by their effect, they have never been separated from the serum. The thermostabile substance, or amboceptor, as it is generally called, has in itself no destructive action on the bacteria; but in some way so alters them that they can be acted on by the thermolabile substance called complement whose action is destructive. The amount of amboceptor may increase in the course of infection and its formation stimulated, the amount of complement remains unchanged. The action of the amboceptor is specific, that is, directed against a single species of bacterium only; the destructive power of the blood may be very great against a single bacterium species and have no effect on others. There seem naturally to be many different amboceptors in the blood, and the number may be very greatly increased. It has been shown as a result of the work of many investigators that the shield has two faces,--there is destruction both by cells and fluids and there is interaction by both. The amboceptors so necessary for the destructive action of the serum are produced by the body cells, particularly the leucocytes. The serum assists in pagocytosis by the action on bacteria of substances called opsonins which are contained in it, and the formation of which can be very greatly stimulated. Again, not all inclusion of bacteria within leucocytes is indicative of phagocytosis; in many cases the bacteria seem to find the best conditions for existence within the leucocytes, and these and not the bacteria are destroyed.

So far it has been shown that the best defence of the body is, as is the best defence in war, by offensive measures, as illustrated by phagocytosis and destruction by the serum. Both of these actions can be increased by their exercise just as the strength of muscular contraction can be increased by exercise, and the facility for doing everything increased by habit. Certain of the infectious diseases are, as has been said, essentially toxic in their nature, and in cultures the organisms produce poisonous substances. By the injection into the tissues of such substances the same disturbances are produced as when the bacteria are injected. Such a disease is diphtheria. In this there is only a superficial invasion of the tissues. The diphtheria bacilli are located on the surface of the tonsils or pharynx or windpipe, where, as a result of their action, the membrane so characteristic of the disease is produced. The membrane may be the cause of death when it is so extensively formed as to occlude the air passages, but the prominent symptoms of the disease, the fever, the weakness of the heart and the great prostration are due not to the presence of the membrane, but to the action of toxic substances which are formed by the bacteria growing in the superficial lesions and absorbed. Tetanus, or lockjaw, is another example of these essentially toxic diseases. The body must find some means of counteracting or destroying these injurious toxic substances. It does this by forming antagonistic substances called antitoxines, which act not by destroying the toxines, but by uniting with them, the compound substance being harmless. It has been found that the production of antitoxine can be so stimulated by the injection of toxine that the blood of the animal used for the purpose contains large amounts of antitoxine. The horse is used in this way to manufacture antitoxine, and the serum injected into a patient with diphtheria has a curative action, a greater amount being thus introduced than the patient can manufacture.

[Illustration: FIG. 18.--DIAGRAM TO ILLUSTRATE EHRLICH'S THEORY OF ANTITOXINE FORMATION. The surface of the cell (_n_) is covered with receptors some of which (_b_) fit the toxine molecule, (_a_) allowing the toxine to act upon the cell. Under the stimulus of this the cell produces these receptors in excess which enter into the blood and there combine with the toxine as in _a^1 b^1_, thus anchoring it and preventing it from acting upon the cells. The receptors c and d do not fit the toxine molecule.]

A very ingenious theory which well accords with the facts has been given by Ehrlich in explanation of the production of antitoxine and of the reaction between toxine and antitoxine (Fig. 18). This is based on the hypothesis, which is in accord with all facts and generally accepted, that the molecules which enter into the structure of any chemical substance have in each particular substance a definite arrangement, and that in a compound substance each elementary substance entering into the compound molecule has chemical affinities, most of which may be satisfied by finding a suitable mate. Ehrlich assumes that the very complex chemical substances which form the living cells have many unsatisfied chemical affinities, and that it is due to this that molecules of substances adapted for food can enter the cells and unite with them; but there must be some coincidence of molecular structure to enable the union to take place, the comparison being made of the fitting of a key into a lock. The toxines--that produced by the diphtheria bacillus being the best example--are substances whose molecular structure enables them to combine with the cells of the body, the combination being effected through certain chemical affinities belonging to the cells termed receptors. Unless the living cells have receptors which will enable the combination with the toxine to take place, no effect can be produced by the toxine and the cells are not injured. This is the case in an animal naturally immune to the action of the diphtheria bacillus or its toxines. In the case of the susceptible animal the receptors of the cells of the different organs combine with the toxine to a greater or less extent, which explains the fact that different degrees of injury are produced in the different tissues; the toxine of tetanus, or lockjaw, for example, combines by preference with the nervous tissue, that of diphtheria with the lymphatic tissue. It is known that in accordance with the general law of injury and repair, a loss in any part of the body stimulates the tissue of the same kind to new growth and the loss is thus repaired; it is assumed that the cell receptors which combine with the toxine are lost for the cell which then produces them in excess. The receptors so produced pass into the blood, where they combine with the toxine which has been absorbed; the combination is a stable one, and the toxine is thus prevented from combining with the tissue cells. The antitoxine which is formed during the disease, and the production of which in the horse can be enormously stimulated by the injection of toxine, represents merely the excess of cell receptors, and when the serum of the horse containing them is injected in a case of diphtheria the same combination takes place as in the case of receptors provided by the patient. In the case of the destruction of bacteria in the blood by the action of amboceptor and complement, the amboceptor must be able to combine with both the bacterial cell and the complement which brings about its destruction, and just as antitoxine is formed so new amboceptors may be formed.

Few hypotheses have been advanced in science which are more ingenious, in better accord with the facts, have had greater importance in enabling the student to grasp the intricacies of an obscure problem, and which have had an equal influence in stimulating research. The immunity which results from disease in accordance with this theory, is due not to conditions preventing the entrance of organisms into the body, but to greater aptitude on the part of the cells to produce these protective substances having once learned to do so. An individual need not practise for many years, having once learned them, those combinations of muscular action used in swimming; but the habit at once returns when he falls into the water.

Infectious diseases and recovery are phases of the struggle for existence between parasite and host, and illustrate the power of adaptation to environment which is so striking a characteristic of living matter.

FOOTNOTES:

[1] The comparison here is with the atrium of a Pompeiian house.

CHAPTER VIII

SECONDARY, TERMINAL AND MIXED INFECTIONS.--THE EXTENSION OF INFECTION IN THE INDIVIDUAL.--TUBERCULOSIS.--THE TUBERCLE BACILLUS.--FREQUENCY OF THE DISEASE.--THE PRIMARY FOCI.--THE EXTENSION OF BACILLI.--THE DISCHARGE OF BACILLI FROM THE BODY.--INFLUENCE OF THE SEAT OF DISEASE ON THE DISCHARGE OF BACILLI.--THE INTESTINAL DISEASES.--MODES OF INFECTION.--INFECTION BY SPUTUM SPRAY.--INFECTION OF WATER SUPPLIES.--EXTENSION OF INFECTION BY INSECTS.--TRYPANOSOME DISEASES.--SLEEPING SICKNESS.--MALARIA.--THE PART PLAYED BY MOSQUITOES.--PARASITISM IN THE MOSQUITO.--INFECTION AS INFLUENCED BY HABITS AND CUSTOMS.--HOOKWORM DISEASE.--INTER-

RELATION BETWEEN HUMAN AND ANIMAL DISEASES.--PLAGUE.--PART PLAYED BY RATS IN TRANSMISSION.--THE PRESENT EPIDEMIC OF PLAGUE.

The infectious diseases are often complicated by secondary infections, some other organism finding opportunity for invasion in the presence of the injuries produced in the primary disease. In many diseases, such as diphtheria, scarlet fever and smallpox, death is frequently due to the secondary infection. The secondary invaders not only find local conditions favoring a successful attack, but the activity of the tissue cells on which the production of protective substances essentially depends has suffered by the primary infection, or the cells are occupied in meeting the exigencies of this. The body is in the position of a state invaded by a second power where all its forces and resources are engaged in repelling the first attack.

What are known as terminal infections occur shortly before death. No matter what the disease which causes death, in the last hours of life the body usually becomes invaded by organisms which find their opportunity in the then defenceless tissues, and the end is often hastened by this invasion.

There are also mixed infections in which two different organisms unite in attack, each in some way assisting in the action of the other. The best known example of this is in the highly infectious disease of swine known as hog cholera. It has been shown that in this disease two organisms are associated,--one an invisible and filterable organism, and the other a bacillus. It was first supposed that the bacillus was the specific organism; it was found in the lesions and certain, but not all, the features of the disease were produced by inoculating hogs with pure cultures. The disease so produced is not contagious, and the contagious element seems to be due to the filterable virus.

The modes of transmission of infectious diseases are of great importance and are the foundation of measures of public health. In the preceding chapter we have seen that in the infected individual the disease extends from one part of the body to another. There is a primary focus of disease from which the extension takes place, and the study of the modes of extension in the individual throws some light on the much more difficult subject of the transmission of disease from one individual to another. There are four ways by which extension in the individual may take place.

1. By continuity of tissue, an adjoining tissue or organ becoming infected by the extension of a focus of infection.

2. By means of lymphatics. Organisms easily enter these vessels which are in continuity with the tissue spaces and receive the exudate from the focus of infection. The organisms are carried to the lymph nodes, which, acting as filters, retain them and for a time prevent a further extension. The following Illustrates the importance of the part the nodes may play in mechanically holding back a flood of infection. A physician examined after death the body of a person who died from infection with a very virulent micrococcus and in the course of the examination slightly scratched a finger. One of the organs of the body was removed, sent to a laboratory and received by a laboratory worker, a woman physician, who had slight abrasions and fissures in the skin of the hands from contact with irritating chemicals. In the course of a few hours the wound on the finger of the man became inflamed, intensely painful, and red lines extended up the arm in the course of the lymphatic vessels, showing that the organisms were in the lymphatics and causing inflammation in their course. The lymph nodes in the armpit into which these vessels empty became greatly inflamed, swollen, and an abscess formed in them which was opened. There was high fever, great prostration, a serious illness from which the man did not recover for several months. The woman only handled the organ which was sent to the laboratory in order to place it in a fluid for preservation. She also had a focus of infection of a finger with the same red lines on the arm, showing extension by the lymphatics; but there was no halt of the infection in the armpit, for all the lymph nodes there had been removed several years before in the course of an operation for a tumor of the breast. A general infection of the blood took place, there was very high fever, and death followed in a few days. The halt of the infection is important in allowing time for the body to make ready its means of defence. One cannot avoid comparing the lymph node with a strong fortress thrown in the path of a victorious invading army behind which the defenders may gather and which affords them time to renovate their strength.

3. By means of the blood. The blood vessels are universally distributed, the smaller vessels have thin walls easily ruptured and easily penetrated. It is probable that in every infection some organisms enter the blood which, under usual conditions, is peculiarly hostile to bacteria. These may, however,

be carried by the blood to other organs and start foci of infection in these.

4. By means of continuous surfaces. The bacteria may either grow along such surfaces forming a continuous or more or less broken layer, or may be carried from place to place in the fluids which bathe them.

All these modes of extension are well shown in tuberculosis. This disease is caused by a small bacillus which does not produce spores, has no power of saphrophytic growth under natural conditions, and is easily destroyed. Moisture and darkness are favorable conditions for its existence, sunlight and dryness the reverse. There are three varieties or strains of the tubercle bacilli which infect respectively man, cattle and birds, and each class of animals shows considerable resistance to the varieties of the bacillus which are most infectious for the others.

The primary seat of the infection in man is generally in the upper part of the lung. The organisms settle on the surface here and cause multiplication of the cells and an inflammatory exudate in a small area. With the continuous growth of the bacilli in the focus, adjoining areas of the lung become affected, and there is further extension in the immediate vicinity by means of the lymphatics. Small nodules are formed and larger areas by their coalescence. Infection with tuberculosis is so common that at least three-fourths of all individuals over forty show evidences of it. The examination of two hundred and twenty-five children of the average age of five years who had died of diphtheria showed tuberculous infection in one-fifth of the cases and the frequency of infection increases with age. The defence on the part of the body is chiefly by the formation of dense masses of cicatricial tissue which walls off the affected area and in which the bacilli do not find favorable conditions for growth. This mode of defence, which is probably combined with the production of substances antagonistic to the toxines produced by the bacilli, is so efficacious that in the great majority of cases no further extension of the process takes place. In certain cases, however, the growth of the bacilli in the focus is unchecked, the tissue about them is killed and becomes converted into a soft semi-fluid material; further extension then takes place. All parts of the enormous surface of the lungs are connected by means of the system of air tubes or bronchi, and the bacilli have favorable opportunity for distribution, which is facilitated by sudden movements of the air currents in the lung produced by coughing. The defence of the body can still keep pace with the attack, and even in an advanced stage the infection can be checked in some cases permanently; in others the check is but temporary, the process of softening continues, and large cavities are produced by the destruction of the tissue. On the inner surface of these cavities there may be a rapid growth of bacilli.

From the lungs the bacilli are carried by the lymphatics to the lymph nodes at the root of the lungs, in which a similar process takes place; this, on the whole, is favorable, because further extension by this route is for a time blocked. The extension by means of surfaces continues, the abundant sputum which is formed in the lungs and which contains large numbers of bacilli, becomes the vehicle of transportation. The windpipe and larynx may become infected, the back parts of each are more closely in contact with the sputum and are the parts most generally infected. A large part of the sputum is swallowed and infection of the intestine takes place, the lesions taking the form of large ulcers. From the intestinal ulcers there is further extension by means of the lymphatics, to the large lymph nodes in the back of the abdominal cavity (Fig. 8-25); the bacilli may also pass from the ulcers into the abdominal cavity and be distributed over the surface of the peritoneum resulting in tuberculous peritonitis. When the disease has reached an advanced stage, bacilli in small numbers continually pass into the blood and are distributed by this over the body, producing small nodules in many places. In rare cases distribution by the blood is the principal method of extension, and immense numbers of small foci of disease are produced, the form of disease being known as acute miliary tuberculosis. Although the bacilli are distributed everywhere, certain organs, as the brain and muscles, are usually exempt, because in these the conditions are not favorable to further growth of the bacilli. Tuberculosis, although frequently a very acute disease, is usually one of the best types of a chronic disease and may last for many years. The chronic form is characterized by periods of slow or rapid advance when conditions arise in the body favorable for the growth of the bacilli, and periods when the disease is checked and quiescent, the defensive forces of the body having gained the upper hand. Often the intervention of some other disease so weakens the defences of the body that the bacilli again find their opportunity. Thus typhoid fever, scarlet fever and other diseases may be followed by a rapidly fatal advance of the tuberculosis, starting from some old and quiescent focus of the disease.

Tuberculosis is also one of the best examples of what is known as latent infection. In this the infectious organisms enter the body and produce primary lesions in which the organisms persist but do not extend owing to their being enclosed in a dense and resistant tissue, or to the production of a local immunity to their action. Dr. Head has recently examined the children of households in which there was open tuberculosis in some member of the household. By open tuberculosis is understood a case from which bacilli are being discharged. He found with scarcely an exception that all the children in such families showed evidences of infection. The detection of slight degrees of tuberculous infection is now made easy by certain skin reactions on inoculation of the skin with a substance derived from the tubercle bacilli. Such latent infections may never become active and in the majority of cases do not. When, however, in consequence of some intercurrent disease or conditions of malnutrition the general defences of the body become weakened extension follows. Such latent infections explain the enormous frequency of tuberculosis in prisons. Under the general prison conditions infection in the prisons probably does not take place to any extent, and the disease is as common when the prisoners are kept in individual cells as in common prisons. It is probable that in these cases the prisoners have latent tuberculosis when entering, and the disease becomes active under the moral and physical depression which prison life entails.

For the extension of infection from one individual to another the infecting organisms must in some way be transferred. The most important of the conditions influencing this are the localization of the disease and the character of the infectious organisms, particularly with regard to their resistance to the conditions met with outside of the body. The seat of disease influences the discharge of organisms; thus, if the disease involve any of the surfaces the organisms become mingled with the secretions of the surface and are discharged with these. If the seat of disease be in the lungs, the throat or the mouth, the sputum forms the medium of extension, which can take place in many ways. The sputum may become dried, forms part of the dust and the organisms enter with the inspired air. The organisms which cause most of the diseases in which the sputum becomes infectious are quickly destroyed by conditions in the open, such as the sunlight and drying; street dust does not play so prominent a part in extension as is generally supposed. Organisms find much more favorable conditions within houses. It is now generally recognized that infection with tuberculosis does not take place in the open, but in houses in which the bacilli on being discharged are not destroyed. The hands, the clothing and surroundings even with the exercise of the greatest care may become soiled with the saliva.

It has been shown that in coughing and speaking very fine particles of spray are formed by the intermingling of air and saliva, which may be projected a considerable distance and remain floating in the air for some time. These particles are so fine as to be invisible; they may be inspired, and their presence in the air forms an area of indeterminate extent around the infected person within which such infection is possible. Such spray formation is also an important means of the extension of infection in the sick individual, for it is continually formed and inspired. It is in this way that the extreme prevalence of broncho-pneumonia in infants and young children is to be explained. No matter what the essential disease, an almost constant finding in young children after death is small areas of inflammation in the lungs in and around the terminations of the air tubes. The situation renders it evident that the organisms which caused the lesions entered the lung by the air tubes. The mouth of the child is unclean and harbors numbers of the same sort of organisms as those causing the lung inflammation; but in the absence of such a mode of infection as is given by spray formation it is difficult to see how the extension from the mouth to the lungs could take place. The weakened condition of the body in these cases favors the secondary infection.

If the disease be located in the intestines, as in typhoid fever and dysentery, the organisms are contained in the fecal discharges, and by means of these the infection is extended. In typhoid fever, dysentery and cholera massive infections of the populace may take place from the contamination of a water supply and the disease be extended over an entire city. One of the most striking instances of this mode of extension was in the epidemic of cholera in Hamburg in 1892. There were two sources of water supply, one of which was infected, and the cases were distributed in the city in the track of the infected supply. Many such instances have been seen in typhoid fever. Certain articles of food, particularly milk, serve as sources of infection. This is more apt to happen when the organism causing the infection grows easily outside of the body. A few such organisms entering into the milk can multiply enormously in a few hours and increase the amount of infectious material. In all these cases the sick individual remains a source of infection, for it is almost impossible to avoid some contamination of the body and the immediate surroundings with the organisms contained in the discharges.

Transmission by air plays but little part in the extension of infection. In such a disease as smallpox, where the localization is on the surface of the body, the organisms are contained in or on the thin epithelial scales which are constantly given off. These are light, and may remain floating in the air and carried by air currents just as is the pollen of plants. There seem to have been cases of smallpox where other modes of more direct transmission could be excluded and in which the organisms were carried in the air over a considerable space. All sorts of intermediate objects, both living and inanimate, such as persons, domestic animals, toys, books, money, etc., can serve as conveyors of infection.

Insects play a most important part in the transmission of disease, and in certain cases, as when a disease is localized in the blood, this is the only means of transmission. There are three ways in which the insect plays the role of conveyor.

1. The insect may play a purely passive part in that its exterior surface becomes contaminated with the discharges of the sick person, and in this way the organisms of disease may be conveyed to articles of food, etc. The ordinary house fly conveys in this way the organisms of typhoid and dysentery. Flies seek the discharges not only for food, but for the purpose of depositing their eggs, and the hairy and irregular surface of their feet facilitates contamination and conveyance. When flies eat such discharges the organisms may pass through the alimentary canal unchanged and be deposited with their feces; they also often vomit or regurgitate food, and in this way also contaminate objects. Flies very greedily devour the sputum of tuberculous patients, and the tubercle bacilli contained in this pass through them unchanged and are deposited in their feces.

[Illustration: FIG. 19.--TRYPANOSOMES FROM BIRDS. All the trypanosomes are very much alike. They contain a nucleus represented by the dark area in the centre and a fur-like membrane terminating in a long whip-like flagellum. They have the power of very active motion within the blood.]

2. Diseases which are localized in the blood are transmitted by biting flies. The biting apparatus becomes contaminated with the organisms contained in

the blood, and these are directly inoculated into the blood of the next victim. The trypanosome diseases form the best example of this mode of transmission. The trypanosomes are widely distributed, exclusively parasitic, flagellated protozoa which live in the blood of a large number of animals and birds (Fig. 19). They may give rise to fatal diseases, but in most cases there is mutual adaptation of host and parasite and they seem to do no harm. One of the most dangerous diseases in man, the African sleeping sickness, is caused by a trypanosome, and the disease of domestic cattle in Africa, nagana, or tsetse fly disease, is also so produced. In certain regions of Africa where a biting fly, the Glossina morsitans, occurs in large numbers, it has long been known that cattle bitten by these flies sickened and died, and this prevented the settling and use of the land. In the blood of the sick cattle swarms of trypanosomes are found. The source from which the tsetse fly obtained the trypanosomes which it conveyed to the cattle was unknown until it was discovered that similar trypanosomes exist in the blood of the wild animals which inhabit the region, but these have acquired by long residence in the region immunity or adaptation to the parasite and no disease is produced. With the gradual extension of settlement of the country and the accompanying destruction of wild life the disease is diminishing. Some of the inter-relations of infections are interesting. The destruction of wild animals in South Africa which, by removing the sources of nagana, rendered the settlement of the country possible was due chiefly to the introduction of another infectious disease, rinderpest, which not only destroyed the wild animals but produced great destruction of the domestic cattle as well.

The sleeping sickness has many features of interest. In the old slavery days it was found that the negroes from the Congo region in the course of the voyage or after they were landed sometimes were affected with a peculiar disease. They were lethargic, took little notice of their surroundings, slept easily and finally passed into a condition of somnolence in which they took no food and gradually died. There was no extension of the disease and it was attributed to extreme homesickness and depression. A similar disease has been known for more than one hundred years on the west coast of Africa, and attracted a good deal of interest and curiosity on account of the peculiar lethargy which it produced and from which it has received the name of "sleeping sickness." Although apparently infectious in its native haunts, it lost the power of spreading from man upon removal to regions where it did not prevail. At first confined to a very small region on the Niger river, it gradually extended with the development of trade routes and the general increase of communications which trade brings, until it prevails in the entire Congo basin, in the British and German possessions in East Africa, and is extending north and south of these regions. The cause of the disease and its mode of conveyance was discovered in 1903. The fly Glossina palpalis which conveys the disease is a biting fly about the size of the common house fly and lives chiefly in the vicinity of water. When such a fly bites an individual who has sleeping sickness its bite can convey the disease to monkeys, on whom the transmission experiments were made. After biting the fly is infectious for a period of two days. After this it is harmless, unless it again obtains a supply of living trypanosomes. There is quite a period in which there are no symptoms of the disease, although trypanosomes are found in the blood and in the lymph nodes, and the individual is a source of infection. The peculiar lethargy which has given the disease its name does not appear until the nervous system is invaded by the parasites. It is impossible to compute accurately the numbers of deaths from this disease--in the region of Victoria Nyanza alone the estimates extend to hundreds of thousands.

3. In the third mode of insect conveyance the insect does not play a merely passive role, but becomes a part of the disease, itself undergoing infection, and a period in the life cycle of the organism takes place within it. In all these cases quite a period of time must elapse before the insect is capable of transmitting the disease; in malaria, which is the best type of such a disease, this period is ten days. Malaria is due to a small protozoan, the _Plasmodium malaria, which was discovered by Lavaran, a French investigator, in 1882. The organism lives within or on the surface of the red blood corpuscles. It first appears as a very minute colorless body with active amoeboid movements, and increases in size, attacks a succession of corpuscles, and finally attains a size as large as or larger than a corpuscle. The corpuscles attacked become pale by the destruction of hemoglobin, swell up and disintegrate, the hemoglobin becoming converted into granules of black pigment inside the parasite. Having attained a definite size the organism forms a rosette and divides into a number of forms similar to the smallest seen inside the corpuscles; these small forms enter other corpuscles and the cycle again begins. This cycle of development takes place in forty-eight hours, and segmentation is always accompanied by a paroxysm of the disease shown in a chill followed by fever and sweating which is due to the effect of substances liberated by the organism at the time of segmentation. A patient may have

two crops of the parasite developing independently in the blood, and the two periods of segmentation give a paroxysm for each, so that the paroxysms may appear at intervals of twenty-four hours instead of forty-eight (Fig. 20). This cycle of development may continue for an indefinite time, and there may be such a rapid increase in the parasites as to bring about the death of the individual; but with him the parasite would also perish, for there would be no way of extending the infection and providing a new crop. The disease has been transmitted by injecting the infected blood into a normal individual.

[Illustration: FIG. 20.--PART OF THE CYCLE OF DEVELOPMENT OF THE ORGANISM OF MALARIA, _a-g_, Cycle of forty-eight hour development, the period of chill coinciding with the appearance of f and g in the blood. The organisms g, which result from segmentation, attack other corpuscles and a new cycle begins. h, The male form or microgametocyte, with the protruding and actively moving spermatozoa, one of which is shown free. i and j are the macrogametes or female forms. k shows one of these in the act of being fertilized by the entering spermatozoa. The differentiation into male and female forms takes place in the blood, the further development of the sexual cycle within the mosquito.]

If a mosquito of the species anopheles bites the affected person, it obtains a large amount of blood which contains many parasites. Within the mosquito the parasite undergoes a further development into male and female sexual forms, which may also form in the blood, termed respectively microgametocyte and macrogamete. From the microgametocyte small flagellate bodies, the male sexual elements microgametes or spermatozoa, develop and fertilize the _macrogametes_; after fertilization this develops into a large body, the _ocyst_ which is attached to the wall of the stomach of the mosquito. Within the ocyst, innumerable small bodies, the sporozoites, develop, make their way into the salivary glands and are injected into the individual who becomes the prey of the mosquito, and again the cycle of development begins. The presence of the parasite within the mosquito does not constitute a disease. So far as can be determined, life goes on in the usual way, and its duration in the insect is not shortened.

The nature of the parasite which produces yellow fever is unknown, for it belongs to the filterable viruses; the infectious material, however, has been shown by inoculation to exist in the blood, and the disease is transmitted by a mosquito of another species, the stegomyia. The development cycle within this takes a period of twelve days, which time must elapse after the mosquito has bitten before it can transmit the disease. Here again the mutual interdependence of knowledge is shown. Nothing could have seemed less useful than the study of mosquitoes, the differentiation of the different species, their mode of life, etc., and yet without this knowledge discoveries so beneficial and of such far-reaching importance to the whole human race as that of the cause and mode of transmission of malaria and yellow fever would have been impossible; for it could easily have been shown that the ordinary culex mosquito played no role. The role which insects may play in the transmission of disease was first shown by Theobald Smith in this country, in the transmission by a tick of the disease of cattle known as Texas fever. The infecting organism pyrosoma bigenimum is a tiny pear-shaped parasite of the red corpuscles. Smith's investigations on the disease, published in 1893, is one of the classics in medicine, and one of the few examples of an investigation which has not been changed or added to by further work.

One of the most interesting methods of extension of infection, showing on what small circumstances infection may depend, is seen in the case of the hookworm disease, which causes such devastation in the Southern States. The organism which produces the disease, the Uncinaria, belongs to the more highly developed parasites, and is a small round worm one-third of an inch long. The worms which inhabit the intestines have a sharp biting mouth by which they fasten themselves to the mucous membrane and devour the blood. The most prominent symptom of the disease is anemia, or loss of blood, due not only to the direct eating of the parasite, but to bleeding from the small wounds caused by its bite. Large numbers of eggs are produced by the parasite which are passed out with the feces, which becomes the only infectious material. In a city provided with water-closets and a system of sewerage there would be no means of extension of infection. The eggs in the feces in conditions of warmth and moisture develop into small crawling larv?which can penetrate the skin, producing inflammation of this, known in the region as the ground itch. The larv?enter the circulation and are carried to the lungs, where they perforate the capillaries and reach the inner surface; from this they pass along the windpipe, and then by way of the gullet and stomach reach their habitat, the small intestine. Unfortunately, the habits and poverty of the people in every way facilitate the extension of the infection. There is no proper disposal of the feces, few of the houses have even a privy attached to them, and the feces are distributed in the vicinity of the houses. This leads to contamination of the soil over wide areas. Most of the inhabitants of the country go barefoot the greater part of the year, and this gives ready means of contact with the larv?which crawl over the surface of the ground. The disease is necessarily associated with poverty and ignorance, the amount of blood is reduced to a low point, and industry, energy and ambition fall with the blood reduction; the schools are few and inefficient; the children are backward, for no child can learn whose brain cells receive but a small proportion of the necessary oxygen; and a general condition of apathy and hopelessness prevails in the effected communities. The control of the disease depends upon the disinfection of the feces, or at least their disposal in some hygienic method, the wearing of shoes, and the better education of the people, all of which conditions seem almost hopeless of attainment. The infection is also extended by means of the negroes who harbor the parasite, but who have acquired a high degree of immunity to its effects and whose hygienic habits are even worse than those of the whites. The organism was probably imported with the negroes from Africa and is one of the legacies of slavery.

The diseases of animals are in many ways closely linked with those of man. In the case of the larger parasites, such as the tapeworms and the trichina, there is a direct interchange of disease with animals, certain phases of the life cycle of the organisms are passed in man and others in various of the domestic animals. A small inconspicuous tapeworm inhabits the intestine of dogs and seems to produce no ill effects. The eggs are passed from the dog, taken into man, and result in the formation of large cystic tumors which not infrequently cause death. Where the companionship between dog and man is very close, as in Iceland, the cases are numerous.

Most of the diseases in animals caused by bacteria and protozoa are not transmitted to man, but there is a conspicuous exception. Plague is now recognized as essentially an animal disease affecting rats and other small rodents, and from these the disease from time to time makes excursions to the human family with dire results. The greatest epidemics of which we have any knowledge are of plague. In the time of Justinian, 542 B.C., a great epidemic of plague extended over what was then regarded as the inhabited earth. This pandemic lasted for fifty years, the disease disappeared and appeared again in many places and caused frightful destruction of life. Cities were depopulated, the land in many places reverted to a wilderness, and the works of man disappeared. The actual mortality cannot be known, but has been estimated at fifty millions. Plague played a large part in the epidemics of the Middle Ages. An epidemic started in 1346 and had as great an extension as the Justinian plague, destroying a fourth of the inhabitants of the places attacked; and during the fifteenth and sixteenth and seventeenth centuries the disease repeatedly raised its head, producing smaller and greater epidemics, the best known of which, from the wonderful description of De Foe, is that of London in 1665, and called the Black Death. Little was heard of the disease in the nineteenth century, although its existence in Asia was known. In 1894 it appeared in Hong Kong, extended to Canton, thence to India, Japan, San Francisco, Mexico, and, in fact, few parts of the tropics or temperate regions of the earth have been free from it. Mortality has varied greatly, being greatest in China and in India; in the last the estimate since 1900 is seven million five hundred thousand deaths. The disease is caused by a small bacillus discovered in 1894 which forms no spores and is easily destroyed by sunlight, but in the dark is capable of living with undiminished virulence for an indefinite time. The disease in man appears in two forms, the most common known as bubonic plague, from the great enlargement of the lymph nodes, those of the groin being most frequently affected. The more fatal form is known as pneumonic plague, and in this the lungs are the seat of the disease.

In the old descriptions of the disease it was frequently mentioned that large numbers of dead rats were found when it was prevalent, and the most striking fact of the recent investigations is the demonstration that the infection in man is due to transference of the bacillus from infected rats. There are endemic foci of the disease where it exists in animals, the present epidemic having started from such a focus in Northern China, in which region the Tarabagan, a small fur-bearing animal of the squirrel species, was infected. Rats are easily infected, the close social habits of the animal, the vermin which they harbor, and the habits of devouring their dead fellows favor the extension of infection. The disease extends from the rat to man chiefly by means of the fleas which contain the bacilli, and in cases of pneumonic plague from man to man by means of sputum infection. The disease once established in animals tends to remain, the virus being kept alive by transmission from animal to animal, and the persistence of the infection is favored by mild and chronic cases.

CHAPTER IX

DISEASE CARRIERS.--THE RELATION BETWEEN SPORADIC CASES OF INFECTIOUS DISEASE AND EPIDEMICS.--SMALLPOX.--CEREBRO-SPINAL MENINGITIS.--POLIOMYELITIS.--VARIATION IN THE SUSCEPTIBILITY OF INDIVIDUALS.--CONDITIONS WHICH MAY INFLUENCE SUSCEPTIBILITY.-- RACIAL SUSCEPTIBILITY.--INFLUENCE OF AGE AND SEX.--OCCUPATION AND ENVIRONMENT.--THE AGE PERIOD OF INFECTIOUS DISEASES.

We have seen that insects serve as carriers of disease in two ways: in one, by becoming contaminated with organisms they serve as passive carriers, and in the other they undergo infection and form a link in the disease. The more recent investigations of modes of transmission of infectious diseases have shown that man, in addition to serving while sick as a source of infection, may serve as a passive carrier in two ways. For infection to take place not only must the pathogenic organism be present, but it must be able to overcome the passive and active defences of the body and produce injury. Pathogenic organisms may find conditions favorable for growth on the surfaces of the body, and may live there, but be unable to produce infection, and the individual who simply harbors the organisms can transmit them to others. Such an individual may be a greater source of infection than one with the disease, because there is no suspicion of danger. The organisms which thus grow on the surfaces have in some cases been shown to be of diminished virulence, but in others have full pathogenic power. Such passive carriers of infection have been found for a number of diseases, as cerebro-spinal meningitis, diphtheria, poliomyelitis and cholera. In all these cases the organisms are most frequently found in those individuals who have been exposed to infection as members of a family in which there have been cases of disease. The other sort of carrier has had and overcome the disease, but mutual relations have been established with the organism which continues to live in the body cavity. Diphtheria bacilli usually linger in the throat after convalescence is established, and until they have disappeared the individual is more dangerous than one actually sick with the disease. Health officers have recognized this in continuing the quarantine against the disease until the organism disappears. In typhoid fever bacilli may remain in the body for a long time and be continually discharged, as in the well-known case of "typhoid Mary."[1]

Single cases of certain infectious diseases may appear in a community year after year, and at intervals the cases become so numerous that the disease is said to be epidemic. Such a disease is smallpox. This is a highly infectious disease, towards which all mankind is susceptible. Complete protection against the disease can be conferred by Jenner's discovery of vaccination. The disease becomes modified when transferred to cattle, producing what is known as cowpox, in which vesicles similar to those of smallpox appear on the skin. The inoculation of man with the contents of such a vesicle produces a mild form of disease known as vaccinia, which protects the individual from smallpox. This protection is fully as adequate as that produced by an attack of smallpox, and we are warranted in saying that if thorough vaccination, or the inoculation with vaccinia, were carried out smallpox would disappear. There are great difficulties in the way of carrying out effective vaccination of the whole population, which are accentuated by the active opposition of people who are ignorant and wilfully remain so. There exists in every state a number of people unprotected by vaccination, and among these single cases of smallpox appear. The unprotected individuals gradually increase in number, forming an inflammable material awaiting the spark or infection which produces a conflagration in the one case and an epidemic in the other.

Cerebro-spinal meningitis is another example of a disease which exists in sporadic and epidemic form. This disease is caused by a small micrococcus, the organisms joined in pairs. The seat of the disease is in the meninges or membranes around the brain and spinal cord. The micrococci enter the body from the throat and nose, and either pass directly from here into the meninges, or they enter into the blood and are carried by this into the meninges. The organisms are easily destroyed and cannot long survive the conditions outside the body, so that for infection to take place the transmission must be very direct. Carriers who have the organisms in the throat, but who do not have the disease, are the principal agents in dissemination. The mortality is high, and even in recovery permanent damage is often done to the brain or to the organs of special sense. Sporadic cases constantly occur in small numbers, and it is difficult or impossible to trace any connection between these cases. At varying intervals, often twenty years intervening, an epidemic appears which sometimes remains local in a city or state, sometimes extends to adjoining cities or states, and may even extend over a very large area. In the epidemics the mortality is much higher than in the sporadic cases. The same explanation given for smallpox cannot apply here, for there is not a similar accumulation of susceptible material. We know there is a great deal of variation in the virulence of the different pathogenic organisms, and the virulence can be artificially increased and diminished. In epidemics of meningitis the virulence of the organisms is increased, as is shown by the greater mortality. It is highly probable that such epidemics are due to changes which arise in the organisms from causes we do not know and which increase their capacity for harm. It is possible that such a change would convert a carrier into a case of disease, the organism acquiring greater powers of invasion. Such a strain of organisms arising in one place and producing an epidemic could be transported to another locality and exert the same action, or similar changes in the organisms could arise simultaneously in a number of places. Analogies to such conditions are given in plants. In certain plants it has been shown that from unknown causes there appears a tendency to the production of variations. A very beautiful herbaceous peony known as "Bridesmaid" after having grown for a number of years in single form, in one year wherever grown suddenly became double. The peculiar thing with the lower unicellular organisms is that the changes which so arise do not tend to become permanent, the organism reverts to its usual character, the disease to its sporadic type.

A very fatal form of poliomyelitis has for a number of years prevailed in Sweden. In the United States there have been continually a number of single cases of the disease, and it is not impossible that a more pathogenic strain of the organism has developed in Sweden and has been imported into this country, giving rise to the much greater extension of the disease in a number of places.

The most cursory study of the infectious diseases shows that there is great variation in the susceptibility of individuals. Even in the most severe epidemics all are not equally affected, some escape the infection, others have the disease lightly, others severely, some die. Chance enters into this, but plays a small part, for the same varying individual susceptibility is shown experimentally. If a given number of animals of the same species, age and weight, even those from the same litter, be inoculated with a given number of bacteria shown to be pathogenic for that species, the results differ. If the dose be necessarily fatal, death will take place at intervals; if a dose smaller than the fatal be used, some animals will die, others will recover. The defences of the organism being centred in the activity of the living tissue, any condition which depresses cell activity may have an effect in increasing susceptibility to infection. Animals which ordinarily are not susceptible to infection with a certain organism may be made so by prolonged hunger, or fatigue, by the influence of narcotics, by reduction of the body temperature, by loss of blood. In man prolonged fatigue, cold, the use of alcohol to excess and even psychic depression increases susceptibility. It has been shown that such conditions are accompanied by a diminution in the power of the blood to destroy bacteria.

There is variation in the susceptibility to infection in the different races of man. If a race be confined to one habitat with close intercourse between the people, such a race may acquire a high degree of immunity to local diseases by a gradual weeding out of the individuals who are most susceptible. A degree of comparative harmony may be gradually established between host and parasite, as is the case in wild animals. These have few diseases, the weak die, the resistant breed; they harbor, it is true, large numbers of parasites, but there is mutual adjustment between parasite and host. Diseases in animals greatly increase under the artificial conditions of domestication. Certain highly specialized breeds of cattle, as the Alderneys, are much more susceptible to tuberculosis than the less specialized. The high development of the variation which consists in a marked ability to produce milk fat is probably combined with other qualities, shown in diminished resistance to disease, and under natural conditions the variation would not have persisted. The introduction of a new disease into an isolated people has often been attended with dire consequences. It is much the same thing with the introduction of disease of plants. In Europe the brown-tail moth and the gypsy moth produce continuously a certain amount of damage to the trees, but their parasitic enemies have developed with them and check their increase. These pests were brought to this country in which there were no conditions retarding their increase and have produced great damage.

It is very difficult to estimate the degree of racial susceptibility. The negro race seems to be more susceptible to certain diseases, such as tuberculosis and smallpox, less so to others, as yellow fever, malaria and uncinariasis. What are apparently differences in susceptibility may be explained by racial customs. A statistical inquiry into death in India from poisonous snakes might be interpreted as showing a marked resistance on the part of the white to the action of the venom, but it is merely a question of the boots of the whites and the naked feet and legs of the natives. The relatively greater frequency of smallpox in the blacks is due to the greater difficulties in carrying out vaccination measures among them and the greater opportunity for infection which results from their less hygienic life. It has always been noted that when plague prevails in Oriental cities, the natives are more frequently attacked than are Europeans. This does not depend upon differences in susceptibility, but on the better hygienic conditions of the whites which prevent the close relation to rats and vermin by which infection is extended. There would be but little extension of the hookworm disease in a community where shoes were worn and the habits were cleanly.

It is by no means improbable that the formation of the habits of civilization was influenced by infection. Most of these habits, such as personal cleanliness, the avoidance of close contact, the demand for individual utensils for eating and drinking, are all of distinct advantage in opposing infection. Certain habits, on the other hand, such as kissing, which probably represents the extension of a habit of sexual origin, are disadvantageous and infection is often transmitted in this way. In syphilitic infection the mouth forms one of the most common localizations of the disease and may contain the causal organisms in great numbers. This, the _spiroch 鎰 a pallida_, is an organism of great virulence, and man is the most susceptible animal. The disease, like gonorrhoea, is essentially a sexual disease, the primary location is in the sexual organs, and it is transmitted chiefly by sexual contact. Of all the infectious diseases, it is the one most frequently transmitted to the unborn child; in certain cases the disease is transmitted, in others the developing foetus may be so injured by the toxic products of the disease that various imperfections of development result, as is shown in deformities, or in conditions which render the entire organism or individual organs, particularly the nervous system, more susceptible to injury. Following the primary localization of the acquired form of the disease, there is usually secondary localization in the mucous membrane of the mouth, and the disease may be transmitted by kissing or by the use of contaminated utensils. The habit of indiscriminate kissing is one which might with great benefit be given up.

There is definite relation between age and the infectious diseases. In general, susceptibility is increased in the young; young animals can be successfully inoculated with diseases to which the adults of the species are immune, and certain human diseases, such as scarlet fever, measles and whooping cough, seem to be the prerogatives of the child. It must be remembered, however, that one attack of these diseases confers a strong and lasting immunity and children represent a raw material unprotected by previous disease. Where measles has been introduced into an island population for the first time, all ages seem equally susceptible. All ages are equally susceptible to smallpox, and yet in the general prevalence of the disease in the prevaccination period it was almost confined to children, the adults being protected by a previous attack. The habits and environment at different ages have an influence on the opportunities for infection. There is comparatively little opportunity for infection during the first year, in which period the infant is nursed and has a narrow environment within which infection is easily controlled. With increasing years the opportunities for infection increase. When the child begins to move and crawl on hands and knees the hands become contaminated, and the habit of putting objects handled into the mouth makes infection by this route possible. Food also becomes more varied, milk forms an important part of the diet, and we are now appreciating the possibilities of raw milk in conveying infection. With the enlarging environment, with the school age bringing greater contact of the child with others, there come greater opportunities for infection which are partly offset by the increase in cleanliness. The dangers of infection in the school period are now greatly lessened by medical inspection and care of the school children. In the small epidemic of smallpox which prevailed in Boston from 1881 to 1883, there was a sharp decline in the incidence of the disease in children as soon as the school age was reached, this being due to the demand of vaccination as a condition for entrance into the schools. Many of the infectious diseases are much milder in children than in adults. This is the case in typhoid fever, malaria and yellow fever. The comparative immunity of the natives to yellow fever in regions where this prevails seems to be due to their having acquired the disease in infancy in so mild a form that it was not recognized as such.

The infectious diseases are preeminently the diseases of the first third of life. After the age of forty man represents a select material. He has acquired immunity to many infections by having experienced them. Habits of life have become fixed and there is a general adjustment to environment. The only infectious disease which shows no abatement in its incidence is pneumonia, and the mortality in this increases with age. Between thirty-five and fifty-five man stands on a tolerably firm foundation regarding health; after this the age atrophies begin, the effects of previous damage begin to be apparent, and the tumor incidence increases.

FOOTNOTE: [1] This was the case of a woman, by occupation a cook, whose numerous exchanges of service were accompanied by the appearance of cases of typhoid fever in the families. This became so marked that an examination was made and she was found to be a typhoid carrier and as such constantly discharging typhoid bacilli. She is now isolated.

CHAPTER X

INHERITANCE AS A FACTOR IN DISEASE.--THE PROCESS OF CELL MULTIPLICATION.--THE SEXUAL CELLS DIFFER FROM THE OTHER CELLS OF THE BODY.--INFECTION OF THE OVUM.--INTRA-UTERINE INFECTION.--THE PLACENTA AS A BARRIER TO INFECTION.--VARIATIONS AND MUTATIONS.-- THE INHERITANCE OF SUSCEPTIBILITY TO DISEASE.--THE INFLUENCE OF ALCOHOLISM IN THE PARENTS ON THE DESCENDANTS.--THE HEREDITY OF NERVOUS DISEASES.--TRANSMISSION OF DISEASE BY THE FEMALE ONLY.-- HEMOPHILIA.-- THE INHERITANCE OF MALFORMATIONS.--THE CAUSES OF MALFORMATIONS.--MATERNAL IMPRESSIONS HAVE NO INFLUENCE.-- EUGENICS.

The question of inheritance of disease is closely associated with the study of infection, and the general subject of heredity in its bearing on disease can be considered here. By heredity is understood the transference of similar characteristics from one generation of organisms to another. The formation of the sexual cells is a much more complex process than that of the formation of single differentiated cells, for the properties of all the cells of the body are represented in the sexual cells, to the union of which the heredity transmission of the qualities of the parents is due. In the nucleus of all the cells in the body there is a material called chromatin, which in the process of cell division forms a convoluted thread; this afterwards divides into a number of loops called chromosomes, the number of which are constant for each animal species. In cell division these loops divide longitudinally, one-half of each going to the two new cells which result from the division; each new cell has one-half of all the chromatin contained in the old and also one-half of the cytoplasm or the cell material outside of the nucleus. The process of sexual fertilization consists in the union of the male and female sex cells and an equal blending of the chromatin contained in each (Fig. 22). In the process of formation of the sexual cells a diminution of the number of chromosomes contained in them takes place, but this is preceded by such an intimate intermingling of the chromatin that the sexual cells contain part of all the chromosomes of the undifferentiated cells from which they were formed. The new cell which is formed by the union of the male and female sexual cells and which constitutes a new organism, contains the number of chromosomes characteristic of the species and parts of all the chromatin of the undifferentiated cells of male and female ancestors. As a result of this the most complicated mechanism in nature, it is evident that in a strict sense there can be no heredity of a disease because heredity in the mammal is solely a matter of the chromosomes and these could not convey a parasite. The new organism can, however, quickly become diseased and, by the transference of disease to it and by either parent, there is the appearance of hereditary transmission of disease, though in reality it is not such. The ovum itself can become the site of infection; this, which was first discovered by Pasteur in the eggs of silkworms, takes place not infrequently in the infection of insects with protozoa. In Texas fever the ticks which transmit the disease, after filling with the infected blood, drop off and lay eggs which contain the parasites, and the disease is propagated by the young ticks in whom the parasites have multiplied. The same thing is true in regard to the African relapsing or tick fever, which is also transferred by a tick. In the white diarrhoea of chickens the eggs become infected before they are laid and the young chick is infected before it emerges from the shell. It is highly improbable, and there is no certain evidence for it, that the extremely small amount of material contributed by the male can become infected and bring infection to the new organism. In the cases in which disease of the male parent is transferred to the offspring, it is either by an infection of the female by the male, with transference of the infection from her to the developing organism, or with the male sexual cells there may be a transference to the female of the infectious material and the new organism may be directly infected. No other disease in man is so easily and directly transferred from either parent to offspring as is syphilis, and the disease is extremely malignant for the foetus, usually causing death before the normal period of intra-uterine development is reached.

[Illustration: FIG. 21.--DIAGRAM SHOWING THE RELATION OF THE SEXUAL

CELLS TO THE SOMATIC CELLS OR THOSE OF THE GENERAL BODY. The sexual cells are represented to the left of the line at the bottom of diagram and are black. From the fertilized ovum at the top there is a continuous cell development, with differentiation represented in the cell groups of the bottom row. It is seen that the sexual cells are formed directly from the germ cell and contain no admixture from the cells of the body.]

The mother gives the protection of a narrow and unchanging environment and food to the new organism which develops within the uterus, and there is always a membranous separation between them. Disease of the mother may affect the foetus in a number of ways. In most cases the membrane of separation is an efficient guard preventing pathogenic organisms reaching the foetus from the mother. In certain cases, however, the guard can be passed. In smallpox, not infrequently, the disease extends from the mother to the foetus, and the child may die of the infection or be born at term with the scars resulting from the disease upon it. Syphilis in the mother in an active stage is practically always extended to the foetus. We have said that in an infectious disease substances of an injurious character are produced by bacteria, and such substances being in solution in the blood of the infected mother can pass through the membranous barrier and may destroy the foetus although the mother recovers from the infection.

[Illustration: FIG. 22.--DIAGRAMMATIC REPRESENTATION OF THE PROCESS OF FERTILIZATION. (Boveri.) In the first cell (_a_) the ovum is shown in process of fertilization by the entering spermatozoon or male sexual element. In the following cells there is shown the increase in amount of the male material and the final intimate commingling in g which precedes the first segmentation. g represents a new organism formed by the union of the male or female cell but differing from either of them.]

Living matter is always individual, and this individuality is expressed in slight structural variations from the type of the species as shown in an average of measurements, and also in slight variations in function or the reactions which living tissue shows towards the conditions acting upon it. The anatomical variations are more striking because they can be demonstrated by weight and measure, but the functional variations are equally numerous. Thus, no two brains react in exactly the same way to the impressions received by the sense organs; there are differences in muscular action, differences in digestion;

these variations in function are due to variations in the structure of living material which are too minute for our comparatively coarse methods of detection. In the enormous complexity of living matter it is impossible that there should not be minute differences in molecular arrangement and to this such functional variations may be due. Chemistry gives us a number of examples of variations in the reaction of substances which with the same composition differ in the molecular arrangement. Even in so simple a mechanism as a watch there are slight differences in structure which gives to each watch certain individual characteristics, but the type as an instrument constructed for recording time remains. In the fusion of the chromosomes of the male and female sexual cells, to which the hereditary transmission of the ancestral qualities to the new offspring is due, there are differences in the qualities of each, for the individuality of the parents is expressed in the germ cells, and the varying way in which these may fuse gives to the new cell qualities of its own in addition to qualities which come from each ancestor, and from remote ancestors through these. The qualities with which the new organism starts are those which it has received from its ancestors plus its individuality. The fact that the sexual cells are formed from the early formed cells of the new organism which represent all of the qualities of the fertilized ovum or primordial cell, renders it unlikely that the new offspring will contain qualities which the parents have acquired. The question of the inheritance of characteristics which the parents have acquired as the result of the action of environment upon them is one which is still actively investigated by the students of heredity, but the weight of evidence is opposed to this belief.

In the new organism the type of the species is preserved and the variations from the mean to which individuality is due are slight. We are accustomed to regard as variations somewhat greater departures from the species type than is represented in individuality, but there is no sharp dividing line between them.

Very much wider departures from the species type are known as mutations. Such variations and mutations, like individuality, may be expressed in qualities which can be weighed and measured, or in function, and all these can be inherited; certain of them known as dominant characteristics more readily than others, which are known as recessive. If these variations from the type are advantageous, they may be preserved and become the property of the species, and it is in this way that the characteristics of the different races have arisen. Certain of the variations are unfavorable to the race. The varying predisposition to infection which undoubtedly exists and may be inherited represents such a variation. Tuberculosis is an instance of this; for, while the cause of the disease is the tubercle bacillus, there is enormous difference in the resistance of the body to its action in different individuals. The disease is to a considerable extent one of families, but while this is true the degree of the influence exerted by heredity can be greatly overestimated. The disease is so common that in tracing the ancestry of tuberculous patients it is rare to find the disease not represented in the ancestors. A further difficulty is that the environment is also inherited. The child of a tuberculous parent has much better opportunity to acquire the infection than a child without such an environment [page 167]. Other diseases than the infectious seem to be inherited, of which gout is an example. In gout there is an unusual action of the cells of the body which leads to the formation and the retention in the body of substances which are injurious. Here it is not the disease which is inherited, but the variation in structure to which the unusual and injurious action of the cells is due.

While tuberculosis and gout represent instances in which, although the disease itself is not inherited yet the presence of the disease in the ascendants so affects the germinal material that the offspring is more susceptible to these particular diseases, much more common are the cases in which disease in the parents produces a defective offspring, the defect consisting in a general loss of resistance manifested in a variety of ways, but not necessarily repeating the diseased condition of the parent. In these cases the disease in the parents affects all the cells of the body including the germinal cells, and the defective qualities in the germ cells will affect the cells of the offspring which are derived from these. There is a tendency in these cases to the repetition in the offspring of the disease of the parents, because the particular form of the parental disease may have been due to or influenced by variation of structure. One of the best examples of affection of the offspring by diseased conditions of the parents produced by a toxic agent which directly or indirectly affects all the cells of the body is afforded by alcohol when used in excess. Since drunkenness has become a medical rather than a moral question, a great deal of reliable data has accumulated in regard to it as a factor in the heredity of disease. Grotjahn gives the following examples: Six families were investigated in which there were thirty-one children. In all these families the father and grandfather on the father's side were chronic alcoholics, and in certain of the families drunkenness prevailed in the more remote ancestors. The following was the fate of the children: eight died shortly after birth of general weakness, seven died of convulsions in the first month, three were malformed, three were idiotic, three were feeble-minded, three were dwarfs, three were epileptics, two were normal. In a second group of three families there were twenty children. The fathers were drunkards, but their immediate ancestors were free: four children died of general weakness, three of convulsions in the first month, two were feeble-minded, one was a dwarf, one was an epileptic, seven were normal. In a family in which both father and mother and their ancestors were drunkards there were six children: three died of convulsions within six months, one was an idiot, one a dwarf, and one an epileptic. For comparison there were taken from the same station in life ten families in which there was no drunkenness: three children died from general weakness, three from intestinal troubles, two of nervous affection, two were feeble-minded, two were malformed, fifty were normal. Legrain has studied on a larger scale the descendants of two hundred and fifteen families of drunkards in which there were eight hundred and nineteen children. One hundred and forty-five of these were insane, sixty-two were criminals, and one hundred and ninety-seven drunkards. Of course all this cannot be attributed to alcohol alone. There is first to be considered a probable variation in the nervous system which is expressed in the alcoholic habit; second, the environment consisting in poverty, bad associates, etc., which the alcoholic habit brings; third, the alcohol alone. That defective inheritance so frequently takes the form of alcoholism is largely due to the environment. There has never been the opportunity to study on a large scale the effect of the complete deprivation of alcohol from a people living in the environment of modern civilization. There is a possibility, and even probability, that the defective nervous organization which predisposes to alcoholism would seek satisfaction in the use of some other sedative drug. So complex are all the interrelations of the social system that it would be possible to regard alcohol as an agent useful in removing the defective, were it not for its long-enduring action and its effects on the descendants, procreation not being affected by its use.

Diseases of the nervous system are particularly apt to affect the offspring, and often the inherited condition repeats that of the parents. This is due to the fact that most of the nervous diseases depend both upon intrinsic factors which consist in some defective condition of the nervous system representing a variation, and extrinsic factors due to environment or occupation which make the basal condition operative. The definite relation between alcoholism and insanity is due to alcohol acting not as an intrinsic but an extrinsic factor, bringing into effectiveness the hereditary weakness of the nervous system. The influence of heredity in producing insanity is variously estimated at from twenty-six per cent to sixty per cent of all cases. This great difference in the estimation of the hereditary influence is due to the personal equation of the statistician, and the care with which other factors are eliminated. In the more severe form of the hereditary degeneration the same pathological conditions are repeated in the descendants. In certain cases the severity of the condition increases from generation to generation. According to Morel there may be merely what is recognized as a nervous temperament often associated with moral depravity and various excesses in the first generation; in the second, severe neuroses, a tendency to apoplexy and alcoholism; in the third, psychic disturbances, suicidal tendencies and intellectual incapacity; and in the fourth, congenital idiocy, malformations and arrests of development. There are some very definite data with regard to inheritance in the nervous disease known as epilepsy. The essential condition in this consists in attacks of unconsciousness, usually accompanied by a discharge of nerve force shown in convulsions, the attack being often preceded by peculiar sensations of some sort known as the aura. In the most marked forms of the affection heredity plays but little part, owing to the early supervention of imbecility and helplessness, and it is a greater factor in the better classes of society than in the proletariat. In the better classes, owing to the greater care of the cases and the avoidance of exciting causes of the attacks, the disease is better controlled and rarely advances to the extent that it does among the poor. The association of epilepsy and alcoholism is especially dangerous, for a slight amount of alcohol may greatly accentuate the disease. In five hundred and thirty-five children in whose parentage there were sixty-two male and seventy-four female epileptics, twenty-two were born dead, one hundred and ninety-five died from convulsions in infancy, twenty-seven died in infancy from other causes, seventy-eight were epileptics, eleven were insane, thirty-nine were paralyzed, forty-five were hysterical, six had St. Vitus's dance, one hundred and five were ordinarily healthy. That variations in the nervous system which produce more or less unusual mental peculiarities and which do not take the form of nervous disease are inherited, the most superficial consideration shows. A child in its mental characteristics is said to take after one or the other of its parents, certain habits and mental traits are the same, often even the handwriting of a child resembles that of a parent.

In certain cases the inheritance is transmitted by the female alone. This is the case in the haemophilia, the unfortunate subjects of which are known as bleeders. There is in this a marked tendency to haemorrhage which depends upon an alteration in the character of the blood which prevents clotting. This, the natural means of stopping bleeding from small wounds, being in abeyance, fatal haemorrhage may result from pulling a tooth or from an insignificant wound. There is a seeming injustice in the inheritance, for the females do not suffer from the disease although they transmit it, while the males who have the disease cannot even create additional sympathy by transmitting it.

The most obvious inheritance is seen in the case of malformations. These represent wide departures from the type of the species as represented in the form. There is no hard and fast line separating the slight departures from the normal type known as variations and mutations, from the malformations. Certain of the malformations known as monstrosities hardly represent the human type. These are the cases in which the foetus is represented in a formless mass of tissue, or there is absence of development of important parts such as the nervous system or there is more or less extensive duplication of the body. There has always been a great deal of popular interest attached to the malformations owing to the part which maternal impressions are supposed to play in their production. In this, some striking impression made on the pregnant woman is supposed to affect in a definite way the structure of the child. The cases, for instance, in which a woman sees an accident involving a wound or a loss of an arm and the child at birth shows a malformation involving the same part. There is no association between maternal impressions and malformations, although there have been many striking coincidences. All malformations arise during the first six weeks of pregnancy known as the embryonic period, in which the development of the form of the child is taking place, and during which time there is little consciousness of pregnancy. Maternal impressions are usually received at a later period, when the form of the child is complete and it is merely growing. It must be remembered also that there is neither nervous nor vascular connection between the child in the uterus and the mother, the child being from the period of conception an independent entity to which the mother gives nutriment merely. Of course, as has been said, the mother may transmit to the child substances which are injurious, and in certain cases parasites may pass from the mother to the foetus. The same types of malformations which occur in man are also seen in birds, and it would require a more vigorous imagination than is usual to believe that a brooding hen could transmit an impression to an egg and that a headless chick could result from witnessing the sacrifice of an associate. The idea of the importance of maternal impressions in influencing the character of the offspring is a very old one, a well-known instance being the sharp practice of Jacob's using peeled wands to influence the color of his cattle. In regard to coincidences the great number of cases in which strong impressions made on the mind of the pregnant mother without result on the offspring are forgotten. The belief has been productive of great anxiety and even unhappiness during a period which is necessarily a trying one, and should be dismissed as being both theoretically impossible and unsupported by fact.

The malformations are divided anatomically into those characterized, first, by excess formation, second, by deficient formation, third, by abnormal displacement of parts. They are due to intrinsic causes which are in the germ, and which may be due to some unusual conditions in either the male or female germ cell or an imperfect commingling of the germinal material, and to extrinsic causes which physically, as in the nature of a shock or chemically as by the action of a poison, may affect the embryo through the mother. Malformations are made more numerous in chickens by shaking the eggs before brooding. A number of malformations are produced by accidental conditions arising in the environment; for instance, the vascular cord connecting mother and child may become wound around parts constricting them or even cutting them off, and the membrane around the child may become adherent to certain parts and prevent the development of these. The extrinsic causes are more operative the more unfavorable is the environment of the mother. Malformations are more common in illegitimate children than in legitimate and more common in alcoholic mothers; there is an unfavorable environment of poverty in both cases, added to in the latter and usually in the former by the injurious action of the alcohol.

The more extensive malformations have no effect on heredity, because the subjects of them are incapable of procreation. The malformations which arise from the accidents of pregnancy and which are compatible with a perfectly normal germ are in the nature of acquired characteristics and are not inherited. Those malformations, however, which are due to qualities in the germinal material itself are inherited, and certain of them with remarkable persistence. There are instances in which the slight malformation consisting in an excess of fingers or toes has persisted through many generations. It may occasionally lapse in a generation to reappear later. In certain cases, notably in the bleeders, the inheritance is transmitted by the female alone, in other cases by the sexes equally, but there are no cases of transmission by the male line only. It is evident that when the same malformation affects both the male and the female line the hereditary influence is much stronger. A case has been related to me in which most of the inhabitants in a remote mountain valley in Virginia where there has been much intermarriage have one of the joints of the fingers missing. There is a very prevalent idea that in close intermarriage in families variations and malformations often unfortunate for the individual are more common. All experimental evidence obtained by interbreeding of animals shows that close interbreeding is not productive of variation, but that variations existing in the breed become accentuated. Variations either advantageous or disadvantageous for the race or individual may either of them become more prevalent by close intermarriage. It seems, however, to have been shown by the customs of the human race that very close intermarriage is disadvantageous.

Eugenics, which signifies an attempt at the betterment of the race by the avoidance of bad heredity, has within recent years attracted much attention and is of importance. Some of its advocates have become so enthusiastic as to believe that it will be possible to breed men as cattle and ultimately to produce a race ideally perfect. It is true that by careful selection and regulation of marriage certain variations, whether relating to coarse bodily form or to the less obvious changes denoted by function, can be perpetuated and strengthened. That the Semitic race excels in commerce is probably due to the fact that the variation of the brain which affected favorably the mental action conducive to this form of activity, was favorable for the race in the hostile environment in which it was usually placed and transmitted and strengthened by close intermarriage. It is impossible, however, to form a conception of what may be regarded as an ideal type of the human species. The type which might be ideal in a certain environment might not be ideal in another, and environment is probably of equal importance with the material. The eugenics movement has enormously stimulated research into heredity by the methods both of animal experimentation and observation, and study of heredity in man. As in all of the beginning sciences there is not the close inter-relation of observed facts and theory, but there is excess of theory and dearth of facts. Certain considerations, however, seem to be evident. It would seem to be evident that individuals should be healthy and enabled to maintain themselves in the environment in which they are placed, but the qualities which may enable an individual successfully to adapt himself to factory life, or life in the crowds and strong competition of the city, may not be, and probably are not, qualities which are good for the race in general or for his immediate descendants. At present our attempts to influence heredity should be limited to the heredity of disease only. We can certainly say that intermarriage between persons who have tuberculosis or in whose families the disease has prevailed is disadvantageous for the offspring; the same holds true for insanity and for nervous diseases of all sorts, for forms of criminality, for alcoholism, and for those diseases which are long enduring and transmitted by sexual contact such as syphilis and gonorrhoea. It is of importance that the facts bearing on the hereditary transmission of disease should become of general knowledge, in order that the dangers may be known and voluntarily avoided. No measures of preventive medicine are successful which are not supported by a public educated to appreciate their importance, and the same holds true of eugenics. How successful will be public measures leading to the prevention of offspring in the obviously unfit by sterilization of both males and females is uncertain. It is doubtful whether public sentiment at the present time will allow the measure to be thoroughly carried out. Some results in preventing unfit heredity may be attained by the greater extension of asylum life, but the additional burden of this upon the labor of the people would be difficult to bear. At best such measures would only be carried out in the lower class of society.

CHAPTER XI

CHRONIC DISEASES.--DISEASE OF THE HEART AS AN EXAMPLE.--THE STRUCTURE AND FUNCTION OF THE HEART.--THE ACTION OF THE VALVES.--THE PRODUCTION OF HEART DISEASE BY INFECTION.--THE CONDITIONS PRODUCED IN THE VALVES.--THE MANNER IN WHICH DISEASE OF THE VALVES INTERFERES WITH THEIR FUNCTION.--THE COMPENSATION OF INJURY BY INCREASED ACTION OF HEART.--THE ENLARGEMENT OF THE HEART.--THE RESULT OF IMPERFECT WORK OF THE HEART.--VENOUS CONGESTION.--DROPSY.--CHRONIC DISEASE OF THE NERVOUS SYSTEM.--INSANITY.--

RELATION BETWEEN INSANITY AND CRIMINALITY.--ALCOHOLISM AND SYPHILIS FREQUENT CAUSES OF INSANITY.--THE DIRECT AND INDIRECT CAUSES OF NERVOUS DISEASES.--THE RELATION BETWEEN SOCIAL LIFE AND NERVOUS DISEASES.--FUNCTIONAL AND ORGANIC DISEASE.--NEURASTHENIA.

Chronic diseases are diseases of long duration and which do not tend to result in complete recovery; in certain cases a cause of disease persists in the body producing constant damage, or in the course of disease some organ or organs of the body are damaged beyond the capacity of repair, and the imperfect action of such damaged organs interferes with the harmonious inter-relation of organs and the general well-being of the body. The effect of damage in producing chronic disease may not appear at once, for the great power of adaptation of organs and the exercise of reserve force may for a time render the damage imperceptible; when, however, age or the supervention of further injury diminishes the power of adaptation the condition of disease becomes evident. Chronic disease may be caused by parasites when the relation between host and parasite is not in high degree inimical, as in tuberculosis, gonorrhoea, syphilis, most of the trypanosome diseases and the diseases produced by the higher parasites. In certain cases the chronic disease represents really a series of acute onsets; thus in the case of the parasites there may be periods of complete quiescence of infection but not recovery, the parasites remaining in the body and attacking when the defences of the body are in some way weakened. In such cases there may be temporary immunity produced by each excursion of the disease, but the immunity is not permanent nor is the parasite destroyed. There is a further connection between chronic disease and infection in that the damage to the organs, which is the great factor underlying chronic disease, is so often the result of an infection.

The infectious diseases are those of early life; chronic disease, on the other hand, is most common in the latter third of life. This is due to the fact that in consequence of the general wear of the body this becomes less resistant, less capable of adaptation, and organic injury, which in the younger individual would be in some way compensated for, becomes operative. The territory of chronic disease is so vast that not even a superficial review of the diseases coming under this category can be attempted in the limits of this book, and it will be best to give single examples only, for the same general principles apply to all. One of the best examples is given in chronic disease of the heart.

The heart is a hollow organ forming a part of the blood vascular system and serving to give motion to the blood within the vessels by the contraction of its strong muscular walls. It is essentially a pump, and, as in a pump, the direction which the fluid takes when forced out of its cavity by the contraction of the walls diminishing or closing the cavity space, is determined by valves. The contraction of the heart, which takes place seventy to eighty times in a minute, is automatic and is due to the essential quality of the muscle which composes it. The character, frequency and force of contraction, however, can be influenced by the nervous system and by the direct action of substances upon the heart muscle. The heart is divided by a longitudinal partition into a right and left cavity, and these cavities are divided by transverse septa, with openings in them controlled by valves, each into two chambers termed auricle and ventricle. The auricle and ventricle on each side are completely separated.

The circulation of the blood through the heart is as follows: The blood, which in the veins of the body is flowing towards the heart, passes by two channels, which respectively receive the blood from the upper and lower part of the body, into the right auricle. When this becomes distended it contracts, forcing the blood into the right ventricle; the ventricle then contracts and sends the blood into the arteries of the lungs, the passage of blood into the auricle being prevented by valves which close the opening between auricle and ventricle when the latter contracts upon its contents. When the ventricle empties by its contraction the wall relaxes and the back flow from the artery is prevented by crescentic-shaped valves placed where the artery joins the ventricle. A similar arrangement of valves is on the left side of the heart. The pressure given the blood by the contraction of the right ventricle sends it through the lungs; from these, after it has been oxygenated, it passes into the left auricle, then into the left ventricle and from this into the great artery of the body, the aorta, which gives off branches supplying the capillaries of all parts of the body. Both of the auricles and both of the ventricles contract at the same, time, the ventricular contraction following closely upon the contraction of the auricles. Contraction or systole is followed by a pause or diastole during which the blood flows from the veins into the auricles. The work which the right ventricle accomplishes is very much less than that of the left, and the right ventricle has a correspondingly thinner wall. The size of the heart is influenced by the size and the occupation of the individual being larger in the large individual than in the small, and larger in the active and vigorous than in the inactive. Generally speaking, the heart is about as large as the closed fist of its possessor.

Imperfections of the heart which interfere with its action may be the result of failure of development or disease. An imperfect heart which can, however, fully meet the limited demands made upon it in intra-uterine life, may be incapable of the work placed upon it in extra-uterine life. Children with imperfectly formed hearts may be otherwise perfect at birth, but they have a bluish color due to the imperfect supply of the blood with oxygen, and are known as blue babies. The condition becomes progressively worse due to the progressive demands made upon the heart, and death takes place after some days or months or years, the time depending upon the degree of the imperfection.

Much of the damage of the heart in later life is due to infection. The valves of the heart are a favorite place for attack by certain sorts of bacteria which get into the blood. This is due to the prominent position of the valves which brings them in contact with all the blood in the body, the large extent and unevenness of the surface and to the rubbing together and contact of their edges when closed. At the site of infection there is a slight destruction of tissue and on this the blood clots producing rough wart-like projections. The valves in some cases are to a greater or less extent destroyed, they may become greatly thickened and by the deposit of lime salts converted into hard, stony masses. Essentially two conditions are produced. In one the thickened, unyielding valves project across the openings they should guard, and thus by constricting the opening interfere with the passage of blood either through the heart or from it. In the other the valves are so damaged that they cannot properly close the orifices they guard, and on or after the contraction of the cavities there is back flow or regurgitation of the blood. If, for instance, the orifice of the heart into the aorta is narrowed, then the left ventricle can only accomplish its work of projecting into the aorta a given amount of blood in a given time by contracting with greater force and giving a greater rapidity to the stream passing through the narrow orifice. This the heart can do because, like all other organs of the body, it has a large reserve force which enables it, even suddenly, to meet demands double the usual, and like all other muscles of the body it becomes larger and stronger by increased work. The condition here is much simpler than when the same valve is incapable of perfect closure, or when both obstruction and imperfect closure, are combined as they not infrequently are. In such cases the ventricle must do more than in the first case. It must force through the orifice, which may be narrowed, the amount of blood which is necessary to keep up the pressure within the aorta and give to the circulation the necessary rapidity of flow, and also the amount which flows back into the heart through the imperfectly acting valve. This it can do by contracting with greater force upon a larger amount of blood, the cavity becoming enlarged to receive this. Not only may such damage to the valves be produced, but the muscular tissue of the heart may suffer from defective nutrition or from the effect of poisons, whether these are formed in the body as the effect of disease or introduced from without; or in consequence of disease in the lungs the flow of blood through them may be impeded, or disease elsewhere in the body, as in the kidneys may, by increasing the pressure of the blood within the arteries, throw more than the usual amount of work upon the heart.

The power of the heart in meeting these conditions, however various they are and however variously they act, seems little short of marvellous, and it goes on throwing three and one-third ounces of blood seventy or eighty times a minute into a tube against nine feet of water pressure, working often perfectly under conditions which would be fatal to a machine. As long as this goes on the injury is said to be compensated for; the increased work which the heart is able to accomplish by the exercise of its reserve force and by becoming larger and stronger enables it to cope with the adverse conditions. With increased demand for work there is a gradual diminution of the reserve force. An individual may be able to carry easily forty pounds up a hill and by exerting all his force may carry eighty pounds, but if he habitually carries the eighty pounds, even though the muscles become stronger by exercise the load cannot be again doubled. The dilatation of the heart which is so important in compensation is fraught with danger, because any weakening of the muscle increases the dilatation, until a point is reached when, owing to the dilatation of the orifices between auricles and ventricles, the valves become incompetent to close them.

When the heart is not able to accomplish its work, the effect of the condition becomes apparent by the accumulation of blood within the veins and a less active circulation. This affects the nutrition and the capacity for work of all the organs of the body, and the imperfect function of the organs may in a variety of ways make still greater demands upon an already overloaded heart. Other conditions supervene. The increased pressure within the veins and capillaries due to the impossibility of the blood in the usual amount passing through or from the heart increases the amount of fluid in the tissues. There is always an interchange between the blood within the vessels and the fluid outside of them; the passage of fluid from the vessels is facilitated by the increased pressure within them, just as pressure upon a filtering fluid increases the rapidity of filtration, and the increase of pressure within veins and capillaries impedes passage of tissue fluid into them. The fluid accumulates within the tissues leading to dropsy, or the accumulation may take place in some of the cavities of the body. The diminished flow of blood through the lungs prevents its proper oxygenation; this may also be interfered with by the accumulation of fluid within the air spaces of the lungs.

Every additional burden thrown upon the heart increases the evil. In women the additional burden of pregnancy may suffice to overcome a compensation which has been perfect, and the same may result from an acute attack of disease. Age, diminishing as it does the capacity for work in all organs, diminishes the compensation capacity of the heart, and a heart which at the age of forty acts perfectly may break down at the age of fifty. Compensation may be gained in other ways, as by reducing the demand made upon the heart by changing the mode of life, by leading an inactive rather than an active life, by avoiding excitement or any condition which entails work of the heart. Social conditions are of great importance; it makes a great difference whether the unfortunate possessor of such a heart be a stevedore whose capital lies in the strength of his muscles, or a more fortunately placed member of society for whom the stevedore works and whose occupation or lack of occupation does not interfere with the adjustment of his external relations to the condition of his heart.

Disease of the nervous system does not differ from disease elsewhere. The system is complex in structure and in function. It consists in nerves which are composed of very fine fibrils distributed in all parts of the body and serve the purpose of conduction, and a central body composed of the brain and spinal cord which is largely cellular in character; it receives impressions by means of the nerves and sends out impulses which produce or affect action in all parts. By means of the organs of special sense, the brain receives impressions from the outer world which it transforms into the concepts of consciousness. Many of the impressions which the central nervous system receives from nerves other than those of special sense and even many of the impressions from these and the impulses which it sends out do not affect consciousness. The memory faculty is seated in the brain and all parts of the brain are closely connected by means of small nerve fibres. The nervous system plays an important part in the internal regulation and coordination of all parts of the body, and it is by means of this that the general adjustment of man with his environment is effected.

Malformations of the brain, except very gross conditions which are incompatible with extra-uterine existence, are not very common. At birth those parts of the brain which are the seat of memory and what are understood as the higher faculties are very imperfectly developed. Variations in structure are extremely common, there are differences in different individuals in the nerves and in the number, size, form and arrangement of the nerve cells, and so complex is the structure that considerable variation can exist without detection. The tissue of the central nervous system has a considerable degree of resistance to the action of bacteria, but is, however, very susceptible to injury by means of poisons. Serious injury or destruction of tissue of the brain and spinal cord is never regenerated or repaired, but adjustment to such conditions may be effected by reciprocity of function, other cells taking up the functions of those which were destroyed.

Certain parts of the brain are associated with definite functions; thus, there are areas which influence or control speech and motion of parts as the arm or leg, and there are large areas known as the silent areas whose function we do not know. All activity of the central nervous system, however expressed, is due to cell activity and is associated with consumption of cell material which is renewed in periods of repose and sleep. Fig. 13 shows a nerve cell of a sparrow at the end of a day's activity and the same after the repose of a night.

Diseases of the nervous system have a special interest in that they so often interfere with man in his relations with his fellows. In diseases of other organs the disturbances set up concern the individual only. Thus, others need not be disturbed save by the demands made on their sympathies by an individual with a cold in the head or a cancer of the stomach. Disease of the nervous system is another affair, instead of those reactions and expressions of activity to which we are accustomed and to which society is adjusted, the reactions and activities are unusual and the individual in consequence does not fit into the social state and is said to be anti-social. There are all possible grades of this, from mere unpleasantness in the social relations with such an individual, to states in which he is dangerous to society and must be isolated from it. Insanity is an extreme case. There is no disease signified in the expression, but it is merely a legal term to designate those individuals whose actions are opposed to the social state and who are not responsible for them. In insanity there is falsity in impressions, in conceptions, in judgment, a defective power of will and an uncontrollable violence of emotion. The individual is prevented from thinking the thoughts or feeling the feelings and doing the duties of the social body in the community in which he lives. The insane are out of harmony with their social environment, but not necessarily in opposition to it.

There is no very sharp line between insanity and criminality. The criminal is in direct antagonism to the laws of social life. An insane person may cause the same injury to society as a criminal, but his actions are not voluntary, whereas the criminal is one who can control his actions, but does not. Mentally degenerated persons, however, can be both insane and criminal. Whatever the state of society, this reprobates the actions of one opposed to it; in a society in which it were usual to appropriate the possessions of others or to devour unpleasant or useless relatives, virtue and lack of appetite would be reprobated as unsocial.

The symptoms of insanity or the manner in which the defective action of the brain expresses itself and the various underlying pathological changes vary, and by combining these it has been possible to subdivide insanity into a number of distinct forms. There are both intrinsic and extrinsic causes of insanity. The intrinsic are the structural differences in the brain as compared with the normal or usual, whether these are due to imperfection in development or to defective heredity or to the injury of disease; the extrinsic causes are those which come from without and bring the intrinsic into activity. Syphilis is a frequent cause of insanity, and probably the only cause of the condition known as general paralysis of the insane, acting by means of the injury which it produces in the cortex of the brain. The abuse of alcohol is another fertile cause, but the changes produced in this are not so obvious as in the case of syphilis. Tumors of the brain are not infrequently a cause, and the same is true of infections, even those not located in the brain. How susceptible the brain is to the effects of the toxines of the infectious diseases is shown in the frequency of delirium in these diseases. There is an interesting relation between this and alcoholism. Alcohol abuse may produce injury, but not sufficient to manifest itself under ordinary conditions; when, however, the action of toxic substance is superadded to the effect of the alcohol the delirium of fever is more marked.

Probably of greater importance than the acquired pathological conditions of the brain in producing insanity is a congenital condition in which the nervous system is defective. The most fertile cause of insanity lies in the inheritance; by this it must not be understood that insane parents produce insane offsprings, but that conditions inherited from immediate or remote ancestors appear in a diminished resistance of the nervous system which is sooner or later expressed as insanity. Given such a defective nervous system, extrinsic conditions which would have no effect on another individual or would be felt in different ways may produce insanity. In these cases occupation plays a great role. The excitement and privations of war especially in the tropics and the ennui of camps leads to insanity in soldiers; occupations such as that of the baker in which there is loss of sleep and the mental strain of students can all act in the same way. A woman who gives no sign of nervous defect may become insane under the strain of pregnancy.

Although insanity is determined by the social relations of man, that part of the social organization which is termed Society, and which has been developed by the idle as a diverting game, is a fertile source of nervous disease and even of insanity, affecting particularly females. The strenuosity of the life, the nervous excitement alternating with ennui, the lack and improper times of sleep, the lack of rest and particularly of restful occupation, the not infrequent use of alcohol in injurious amounts, are all factors calculated to make a defect operative. The so-called "coming out" of young girls is an important element in the game, and their headlong plunge into such a life at a period under any conditions full of danger to the nervous system is especially to be reprobated. If we consider the influence of the game in other respects as conducing to lack of moral sense, to alcoholic abuse (for without the seeming stimulation, but which is really the blunting of impressions which alcohol brings, the game would not be possible), to discontent, to mental enfeeblement, it is all bad. Curiously enough the game is one which in all periods has been played by the idle, but its evil influence is greater now than before when it was the game of royalty chiefly, because there are now more people living from the work of others.

The unusual mental action of the insane not infrequently expresses itself by suicide. The analysis of three hundred deaths from suicide showed pathological changes in the brain in forty-three per cent, and when we think that mental disturbances are very often without recognizable anatomical changes after death, the percentage is very large. In another analysis of one hundred and twenty-four suicides forty-four of these were mentally affected to various degrees. Five of the men and seven women were epileptics, in ten of the families there was hysteria, twenty-four of the men and four of the women were chronic alcoholics.

It is extremely difficult at the present time to say whether insanity is increasing. Statistics in all lands giving the numbers committed to insane hospitals show on their face a great increase, but so many factors enter into these statistics that their value is uncertain. There is now an ever-increasing provision for the care of the insane. Owing to the recognition of insanity as a part of nervous disease and its separation from criminality there is no longer the same attempt to conceal it as was formerly the case, and hospitals for the insane are no longer associated with ideas of Bedlam. It is generally believed that modern conditions in the hurry and excitement of life, and the extreme social differences, the greater urban life, the greater extension of factory life, all tend to an increase in insanity, but there is no absolute proof that this is true. We know very little about insanity in the Middle Ages, but the conditions then were not conducive to a quiet life. There prevailed then as now excess and want, luxury and poverty, enjoyment and deprivations, balls and dinner parties and other features of the social game. There were factions in the cities, public executions, not infrequent sieges, scenes of horror, epidemics, famines, and all these combined with religious superstition and the often unjust and cruel laws should have been factors for insanity. There were actual epidemics of insanity affecting masses of the population, as shown in the children's crusade, the Jewish massacres and the dancing mania in the Rhine provinces. Where civilization seems to be the highest, statistics show the most insane, but this most probably depends upon better recognition of the condition and better provision for asylum care.

The so-called functional diseases have a close relation with diseases of the nervous system, for they chiefly concern the reactions of nerve tissue. Disease expressing itself in disturbance of function only, does not seem to fit in with the conceptions of disease which have been expressed, nor can we imagine a disturbance of function which does not depend upon a change of material. Living matter does not differ intrinsically from any other sort of matter; like other matter its reactions depend upon its composition structure[1] and the character of the action exerted upon it. By functional disease there is expressed merely that no anatomical or chemical change is discoverable in the material which gives the unusual reaction. The further our researches into the nature of disease extend, particularly the researches into the physiology and chemistry of disease, the smaller is the area of functional disease. In functional disease there may be either vague discomfort or actual pain under conditions when usually such would not be experienced, and on examination no condition is found which in the vast majority of cases would alone give rise to that impression on the nervous system which is interpreted as pain. In the production of the sensations of disease there can be change at any place along the line, in the sense organs, in the conducting paths or in the central organ. Thus there may be false visual impressions which may be due to changes in the retina or in the optic nerve or in the brain matter to which the nerve is distributed. It is perfectly possible that substances of an unusual character or an excess or deficiency of usual substances in the fluids around brain cells may so change them that such unusual reactions appear. There may be, of course, very marked individual susceptibility, which may be congenital or acquired. The perception of every stimulus involves activity of the nerve cells, and it is possible that the constant repetition of stimuli of an ordinary character may produce sufficient change to give rise to unusual reactions, and this particularly when there is lack of the restoration which repose and sleep bring. We know into what a condition one's nervous system may be thrown by the incessant noise attending the erection of a building in the vicinity of one's house or the pounding of a plumber working within the house, this being accentuated in the latter case by the thought of impending financial disaster. Even the confused and disagreeable sound due to the clatter of high-pitched women's voices at teas and receptions may, when frequently repeated, be productive of changes in the nerve cells sufficiently marked to give rise to the unusual reactions which are evidence of disease.

In the condition known as neurasthenia, which is often taken as a type of a functional disease, the basal and intrinsic cause is activity of the nervous system with the using up of material which is not compensated for by the renewal which comes in repose and sleep. Neurasthenia is one of the common conditions of our civilization, found among children and adults, the poor and rich, the idle and the factory worker; it is rife in the scholastic professions and among those who earn their living by brain work. It seems to be more common in the upper classes and particularly in the women, but this is because these are more subject to medical care and the condition is more in evidence. There are all sorts of symptoms attached to the condition, for the unusual mental action can be variously expressed. The cerebral form has been thus described by a well-known medical writer: "One of the most characteristic features of cerebral neurasthenia is a weary brain. The sensation is familiar enough to any fagged man, especially if he fall short of sleep. Impressions seem to go half into one's head and there sink into a woolly bed and die. Voices sound far off, the lines of a book run into one another and the meaning of them passes unperceived. Doors bang and windows rattle as they never did before; if a shoestring breaks, an imprecation is upon the lips. Business matters are in a conspiracy to go wrong. Letters are left unopened partly from want of will, partly from a senseless dread lest they contain bad news. At night the patient tosses on his bed possessed by all the cares which blacken with darkness. Headache is common, loss of memory is distressing, and in severe cases it is wider and deeper than mere inattention can explain. There is often the torture of acute hearing, or an inability to suppress attention; the hater of clocks and crowing cocks is a neurasthenic." The disease is especially common in the women players of the social game, and its unhappy victims too often seek relief from the nervous irritability which is a common early symptom in still greater nervous excitement. It is a sad commentary on our civilization that one of the means of treatment for these persons which has been found efficacious is to supply them with some restful household occupation such as knitting or plain sewing, and there are institutions which combine refuge from social activities, often called duties, with simple occupation.

FOOTNOTE: [1] By structure as used in this wide sense, there must be understood not merely the anatomical structure, which is revealed by the dissecting knife and microscope, but molecular structure, or the manner in which elements are arranged to form the molecule, as well.

CHAPTER XII

THE RAPID DEVELOPMENT OF MEDICINE IN THE LAST FIFTY YEARS.--THE INFLUENCE OF DARWIN.--PREVENTIVE MEDICINE.--THE DISSEMINATION OF MEDICAL KNOWLEDGE.--THE DEVELOPMENT OF CONDITIONS IN RECENT YEARS WHICH ACT AS FACTORS OF DISEASE.--FACTORY LIFE.--URBAN LIFE.-- THE INCREASE OF COMMUNICATION BETWEEN PEOPLES.--THE INTRODUCTION OF PLANT PARASITES.--THE INCREASE IN ASYLUM LIFE.-- INFANT MORTALITY.--WEALTH AND POVERTY AS FACTORS IN DISEASE.

Certain conditions have arisen in the past fifty years which have profoundly affected the thoughts, the beliefs and the activities of man. Within this period what is generally known as Darwinism, including under this evolution, has developed. Unlike theories which came from philosophical speculation only, the theory of evolution was one which could be subjected to observation and experiment. It freed man's mind from dogmas, it stimulated the imagination, it enlarged the territory in which it seemed possible to extend knowledge by the methods of science, and has resulted in an enormous increase of knowledge. This has been more striking in medical science than elsewhere, and in this of more far-reaching influence. Evolution coincided with another important development. History shows that all great periods of civilization have at their back sources of energy. In the civilizations of the past such sources of energy have come from the enslavement of conquered peoples or from commerce, or more direct forms of robbery, which have enabled a favored class to appropriate for its purposes the results of the work of others. While these sources have not been absent in the development of our civilization, the great source of energy has come from the rapid, and usually wasteful and reckless, utilization of the stored energy of the earth. The almost incredible advance in medical and other forms of scientific knowledge and the utilization of this knowledge is largely due to the greater forces which we have become possessed of.

Disease plays such a large part in the life of man and is so closely related to all of his activities that the changes in this period must have exerted an influence on disease. We have already seen that within the period we have obtained knowledge of the causes of disease and the conditions under which these causes became operative. The mystery which formerly enveloped disease is gone; disease is recognized as due to conditions which for the most part are within the control of man, and like gravity and chemical attraction it follows the operation of definite laws. There has been developed within the period what is known as preventive medicine, which aims rather at prevention than cure, and the resources of prevention are capable of much greater extension.

Have there been new conditions developed within the period, or an increase of existing conditions which can be regarded as disease factors and which counterbalance the results which have come from the knowledge of prevention and cure? There has been an increase of certain factors of immense importance in the extension of disease. These are:

1. The increase in industrialism, involving as this does an increase in factory life. In many ways this is a factor in disease. (_a_) By favoring the extension of infection, particularly in such diseases as tuberculosis. (_b_) The life indoors, and frequently with the combination of insufficient air and space, produces a condition of malnutrition and deficient general resistance. (_c_) The family life is interfered with by the mothers, whose primary duty is the care of home and children, working in factories, and the too frequent conversion of the house into a factory. (_d_) The influence of factory life is towards a loss of moral stamina rendering more easy of operation the conditions of alcoholism and general immorality. How great has been this increase in industrialism, fostered as it has been by conditions both natural and artificially created by unwise legislation, is shown in the figures from the last census. The number of factory operatives increased forty per cent between 1899 and 1909 and the total population of the country in the period between 1900 and 1910 increased twenty per cent. It is probable that the future will see an extension rather than a diminution of mass labor.

2. The increase in urban life is as conspicuous as the increase in industrialism. In 1880, twenty-nine and five-tenths per cent of the population was urban and seventy and five-tenths per cent was rural; in 1910, forty-six and three-tenths per cent was urban and fifty-three and seven-tenths was rural, the increase being most marked in cities of over five hundred thousand inhabitants. Of the total increase in population between 1900 and 1910, seven-tenths per cent was in the cities and three-tenths per cent in the country. City life in itself is not necessarily unhealthy and there are many advantages associated with it. The conditions which have chiefly fostered it are the immigration of people who are accustomed to community life, the

increase in factory life and the increased number of people of wealth who seek the advantages which the city gives them. The city has always been the favored playground for the social game. The unhealthy conditions of city life are due to the crowding, the more uncertain means of livelihood, the greater influence of vice and alcoholism. Prostitution and the sexual diseases are almost the prerogatives of the cities.

3. All means of transportation have increased and communication between peoples has become more extended and more rapid. In the past isolation was one of the safeguards of the people against disease. With the increase and greater rapidity of communication there is a tendency not only to loss of individuality in nations as expressed in dress, customs, traditions and beliefs, but many diseases are no longer so strictly local as formerly--pellagra, for example. Only those diseases which are transmitted by insects which have a strictly local habitat remain endemic, although the region of endemic prevalence may become greatly extended, as is seen in the distribution of sleeping sickness. Diseases of plants and of animals have become disseminated. Any plants desirable for economic use or for beauty of foliage and flower become generally distributed, their parasites are removed from the regions where harmonious parasitic inter-relations have been established, and in new regions the parasites may not find the former restrictions to their growth. There have been many examples of this, such as the ravages of the brown-tail and gypsy moths which were introduced into New England and of the San Jose scale which was introduced into California. There have been many other examples of the almost incredible power of multiplication of an animal or plant when taken into a new environment, removed from conditions which held it in check, as the introduction of the mongoose into Jamaica, the rabbit into Australia, the thistle into New South Wales and the water-plant chara into England.

It is very difficult to say, but it seems as though there is an increasing unevenness in the distribution of wealth, an increase in the number of persons who live at the expense of the laboring class. Mass labor, effective though it be, makes it easier to divert the proceeds of labor from the laborers. The evidence of this is seen in the increase in number and the prosperity of those pursuits which purvey to luxury, as the automobile industry and the florists' trade and the greatly increased scope and activity of the social game. On the other hand, there is an increase in the number of people who are to a greater or less extent dependent upon extraneous aid, evinced among other ways by the increase in the asylum populations. Both these conditions, wealth and poverty, are important disease factors. Tuberculosis is now a disease of the proletariat chiefly. The measures both of prevention and cure can be and are carried out by the well-to-do, but the disease must remain where there are the conditions of the slums. Of all the conditions favoring infant mortality poverty comes first. In Erfurt, a small city of Germany, of one thousand infants born in each of the different classes, there died of the illegitimate children three hundren and fifty-two; of those of the laboring class, three hundred and five; of those in the medium station (official class largely), one hundred and seventy-three; of those in higher station, eighty-nine. The same relation of infant mortality to poverty becomes apparent when estimated in other ways. In Berlin, with an average infant mortality of one hundred and ninety-six per thousand, the deaths in the best districts of the city were fifty-two and in the poorer quarters four hundred and twenty. The effect of poverty is seen particularly in the bottle-fed infants; with natural nursing the child of poverty has almost as good a chance as the child of wealth. From reasons which are almost self-evident, the mortality in illegitimate infants is almost double that of the legitimate. The greater infant mortality in poverty is due to the more numerous children preventing individual care, the separation of the mother from the nursing child in consequence of the demand made upon her earning capacity, and the decline in breast nursing. Wealth is on the whole more advantageous from the narrow point of view of disease than is poverty, but if we regard its influence on the race its advantages are not so evident. Nothing can be worse for a race than that it should die out, and wealthy families have never reproduced themselves. Conditions always tending to destruction are a necessary part of the environment of poverty; wealth voluntarily creates these conditions, and chiefly by the pernicious influence of its amusements on the young.

A new and in many respects a nobler conception of medicine has been developed. Formerly medical practice was almost exclusively a personal service to the sick individual, and measures looking toward the general relief of disease and its prevention received scanty consideration. The idea of a wider service to the city, to the state, to the nation, to humanity rather than the personal service to the individual, is becoming dominant in medicine. This is seen in the establishment of laboratories by boards of health in cities and states in which knowledge obtained by exact investigations can be made of direct service to the people; in the medical inspection of schools and factories; in promulgating laws directed against conditions which affect health, in the extension of hospitals, and in divers other ways. The idea of public service and of returning to the people in an effective way some of the results of their labor also underlies the large donations which have been given for the creation of special laboratories and institutes in which, through research, greater knowledge of disease may be obtained and made available. The researches which have been made on the nutrition of man and the nutritive value of different foods are of great importance, and this knowledge has not yet begun to be applied as it should be.

There seems to be a balance maintained between the restriction of disease by prevention and the increased influence of social conditions which are in themselves factors of disease. Preventive medicine seems to have made possible, by restricting their harmful influence, the increase in industrialism, in urban life, and in the intercommunications of peoples. The most important aid in the future to the influence of preventive medicine must be the education of the people so that the conditions of disease, the intrinsic and the extrinsic causes and the manner in which these act, shall all become a part of general knowledge, and the sympathy of the people with health legislation and their active assistance in carrying out measures of prevention may be obtained. The effect of social conditions on disease must become more generally recognized.

GLOSSARY

ATROPHY--A condition of imperfect nutrition producing diminution in size and loss of function of parts.

BERTILLON--A French anthropologist who devised a system of measurements of the human body for purposes of identification.

BLOOD-PLASMA--The fluid of the blood.

CELL--The unit of living matter. Living things may be unicellular or composed of a multitude of cells which are interdependent. The general mass of material forming the cell is termed cytoplasm. In this there is a differentiated area termed nucleus which governs the multiplication of cells. In the nucleus is a material termed chromatin which bears the factors of heredity.

CHEMOTROPISM--The influence of chemical substances in directing the movement of organisms.

EXUDATE--The material which passes from the blood into an injured part and causes the swelling.

FIBRIN--The gelatinous material formed in the blood when it clots.

HAEMOGLOBIN--A substance which gives the red color to the blood; by means of its ready combination with the oxygen of the air in the lungs this necessary element is carried to all parts of the body.

INFLAMMATION--Literally a "burning"; the changes which take place in a part after injury.

LYMPH--The fluid which is contained in the lymphatic vessels--nodes. Circumscribed masses of cells connected with the lymphatic vessels.

OSMOSIS--The process of diffusion between fluids of different molecular pressures.

SPORE FORMATION--A mode of reproduction in lower forms of life by which resistant bodies, spores, are formed. These have many analogies with the seed of higher plants.

SYMBIOSIS--A mutual adaptation between parasite and host.

TRANSUDATION--The normal interchange of fluid between the blood and the tissue fluids. The material interchanged is the transudate.

TROPISM--The influence of forces which direct the movement of cells.

ULTRA-MICROSCOPE--A form of microscope which by means of oblique illumination renders visible objects so small as to be invisible with the ordinary microscope.

VIRUS--A substance either living or formed by living things which may cause disease.